ENERGY BOOSTER SMOOTHIES

50 ENERGIZING RECIPES TO FIGHT TIREDNESS, FATIGUE AND BOOST YOUR DAILY ENERGY

Amanda Smith

DISCLAIMER

A smoothie is a thick blend of fruits, vegetables, and dairy products that are rich in protein, minerals and vital supplements. You need a smoothie when you don't have time to make meals as it is a Mighty meal replacement that will fill your body with everything it needs on the go.

Who doesn't love smoothies? A whipped mixture of delicious and creamy ingredients will make you feel like you are top of the world.

So Be smart, learn to make a mind boggling smoothie from this ultimate smoothie cookbook and replace boring beverages with colorful and fast to make perfect smoothies.

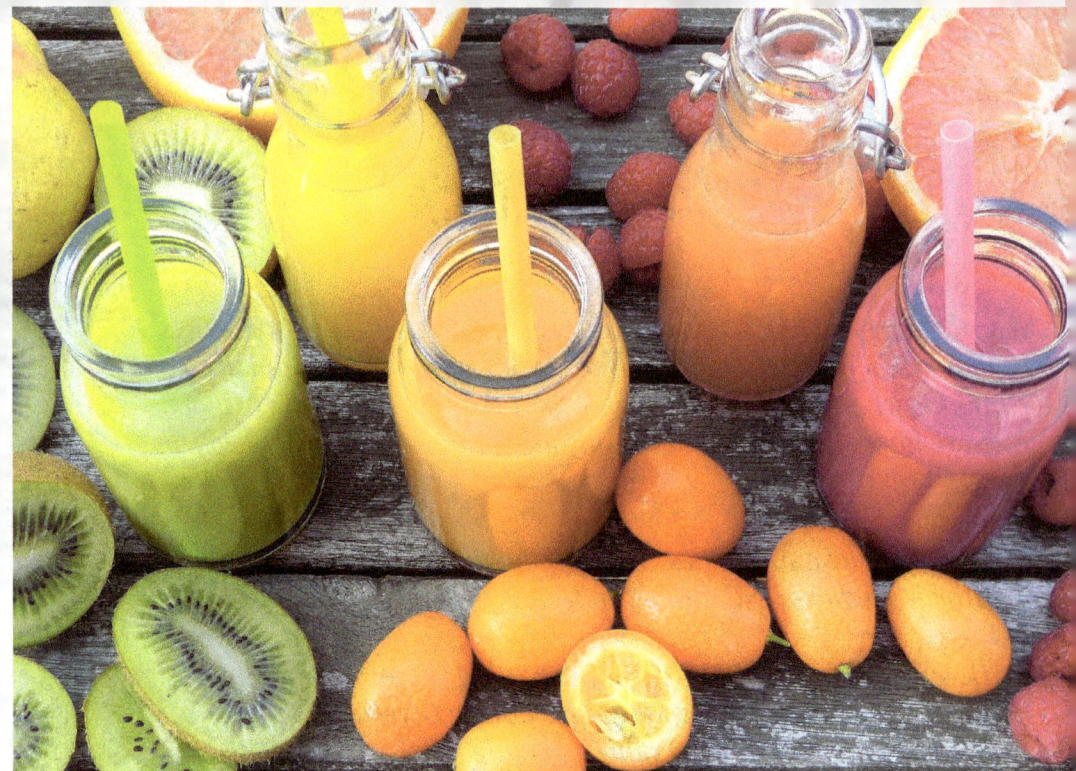

Table of contents

CONTENTS

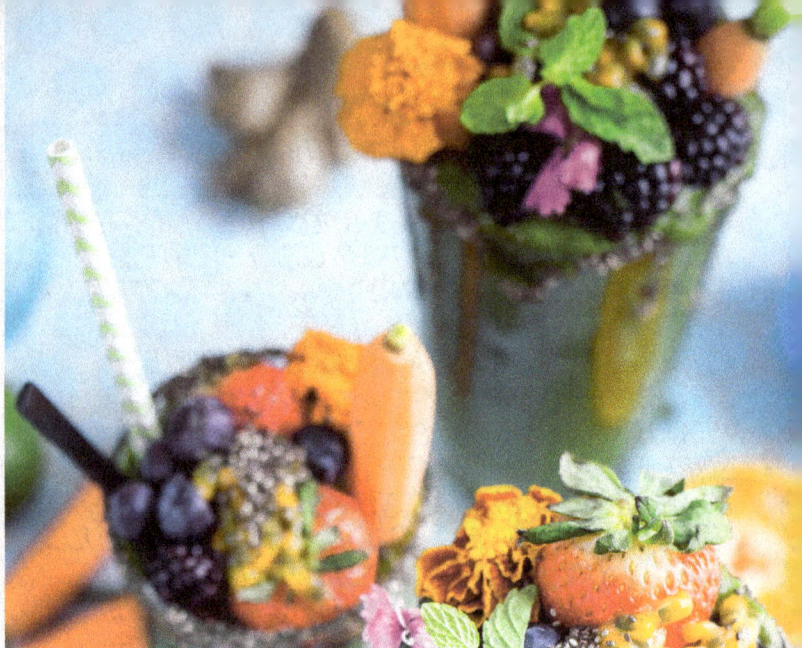

ALL YOU NEED TO KNOW ABOUT SMOOTHIES

"Add a sip of organic, healthy and happy delights to your dreams"

Smoothies are a thickened and blended version of a dairy beverage that has a similar consistency to a shake. They are the pureed form of various combinations of fruit juices, vegetable juices, milk, or even yoghurt. Some smoothies also have various protein powders, multivitamins and other supplements.

People have started consuming smoothies as a part of their meal or even as their meal replacement. Smoothies have now become a demand in the market and are used as an alternative for the replacement of lattes, cappuccinos and other coffee-based drinks.

BASIC COMPONENTS OF A SMOOTHIE

Preparing a smoothie is a diverse task as you may add the ingredients of your choice. But traditionally, most of the smoothies consist of four parts. These 4 parts are:

1. The very first component of a smoothie is a liquid that is considered the base of the smoothie. This base can be either, milk, coconut water or any fruit or vegetable juice.
2. The second component is an assortment of fruits and/or vegetables. These fruits or vegetables are preferably demanded to be frozen. On the other hand, fresh fruits and vegetables can also be used.
3. The third component is the ice that is a considerable component because it helps to retain the thick texture and consistency of the smoothie. Moreover, it enhances the taste of the smoothie as it chills it.
4. The fourth component is the garnishing item or sprinkles that can be either fruit or vegetable chunks being used in the smoothie, or some flavoured powder or sweet sauce.

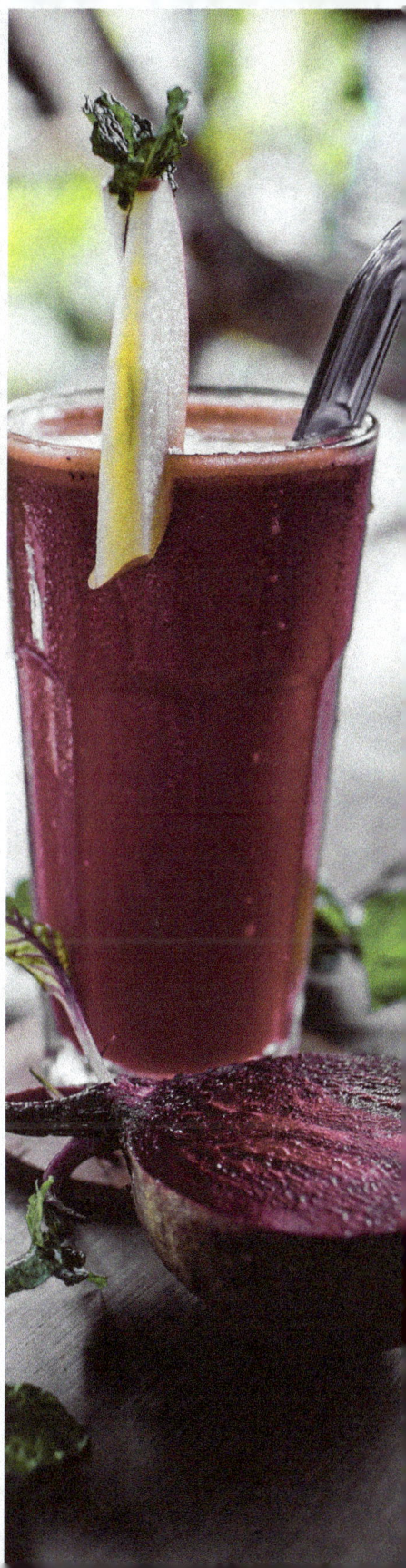

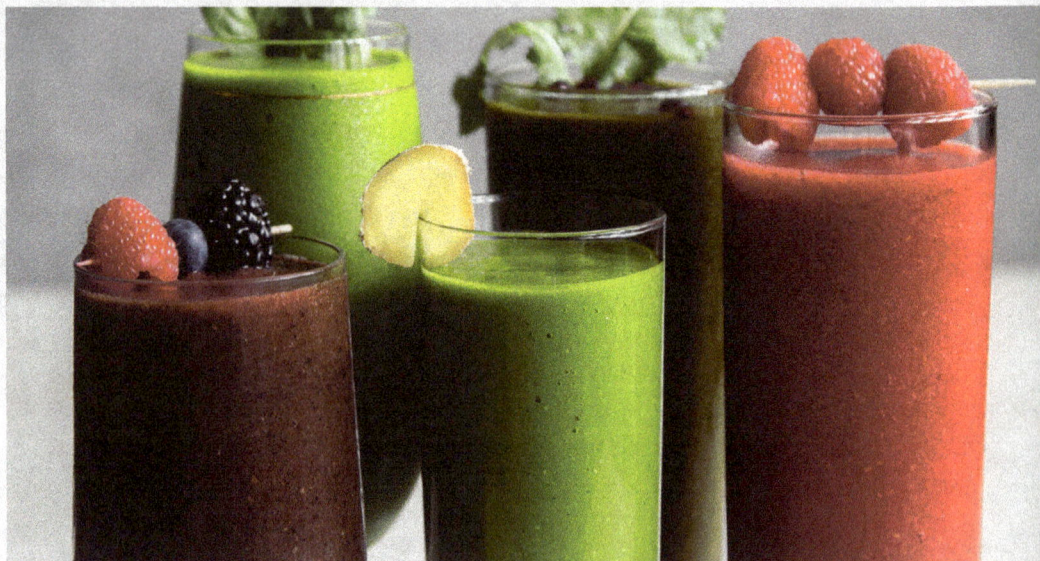

VARIOUS CATEGORIES OF SMOOTHIES

For almost 100 years, people have been making smoothies of their choice. This has led to the development of a variety of smoothies with various ingredients and the way of their preparation. The various recipes can be categorized as:

1. Fruit Smoothies:
These are the smoothies that are made from frozen or fresh fruits. The most popular fruit smoothies are berry smoothies, mango smoothies and banana smoothies. Fruits smoothies have their specificity of being sweet even without using any additional sweetener.

2. Green Smoothies:
Green smoothies are considered to be obtained from green vegetables that's why it is named so. The most popular green smoothies include Kale and spinach smoothie.

3. Nutritious and healthy Smoothies:
The smoothies that are prepared to target nutritional consent, is considered as a healthy smoothie. These smoothies provide the daily RDA of specific vitamins or minerals and aim to replace the supplements and medicines for a particular medical issue. Specific healthy smoothies can be heart-healthy, diabetic-friendly, protein-rich smoothies etc.

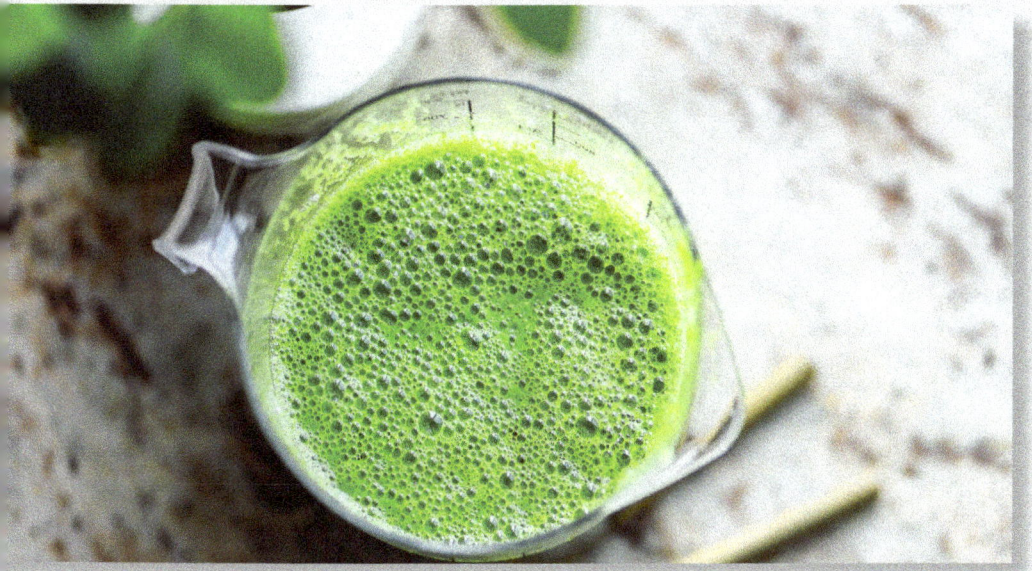

4. Weight Loss Smoothies:

The smoothie with a low glycemic index and no added sugars or sweeteners is the weight loss smoothie. They minimize the carb content and include healthy fats by adding flax seeds or almond butter that help the person to give the feeling of fullness. In weight loss smoothies, green tea, coffee or other caffeine-based stimulants can also be added that not only help to reduce the appetite but also improves the metabolism.

5. Confection Smoothies:

These smoothies are in the form of dessert and contain added sugar, artificial sweeteners and fats that are in the form of ice cream. The confection smoothies are dessert-like beverages having a taste similar to shakes.

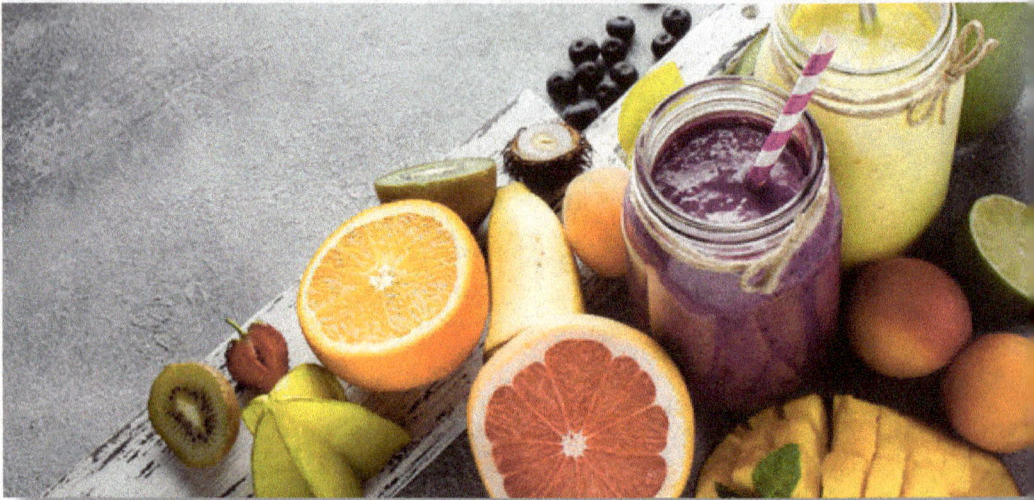

ARE SMOOTHIES PRIOR TO THE JUICES AND SHAKES?

Definitely yes!!
Smoothies contain non-processed, fresh, organic, fruits/vegetables and other items without any artificial sweeteners or syrups. Whereas, shakes contain a large number of processed sugars and ice-creams have been used while preparing the shakes.

On the other hand, juices are the concentrated form of fruits or vegetables and contain the left out juice only. While smoothies are blended mixtures of whole fruits and vegetables with all the original fibre content.

WHY DO YOU NEED SMOOTHIES?

Abundant reasons have convinced the essentiality of smoothies for our health as well as cravings. Smoothies being nutrient-dense, provide you with the maximum dietary intake of your nutritional needs. Despite being delicious and healthy, smoothies can also be a quick meal option with the right fuel for your energy.
Considerably, you need to add smoothies in your life because they can be your immunity and brain booster along with a sense of calm. Smoothies can be your life-changer if made with the right ingredients and using the recommended quantities.
Discussing the benefits of consuming smoothies in your diet will further elaborate its importance.

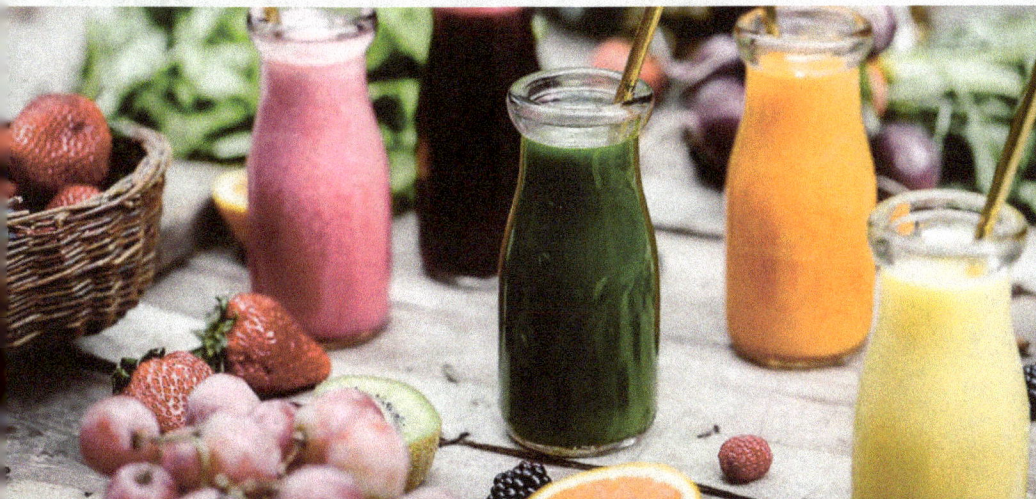

BENEFITS OF CONSUMING SMOOTHIES

1. GUT-FRIENDLY
Increased consumption of green leafy vegetables through the intake of smoothies aids in the digestion process. The high fibre content and the essential vitamins and minerals in these vegetables are the major contributors.

2. IMMUNITY BOOSTER
Smoothies have a good amount of beta-carotene that are helpful for the body to fight against pathogens and health conditions.

3. DETOXIFICATION
Several items like dandelion greens, kale, garlic, papaya and beets can cleanse the body thoroughly. The smoothies are helpful in the removal of toxins that are accumulated within the body tissues.

4. PREVENTS VARIOUS DISEASES
Specific smoothies are introduced to prevent or reduce the chance of a particular disease i.e. heart disease, diabetes, cancer, hypertension etc.

5. STRESS BUSTER
The fresh ingredients used for the preparation of smoothies contain the nutrients that not only boost your energy but also produce happy hormones. Smoothies can even control your mood swings and helps in fighting depression.

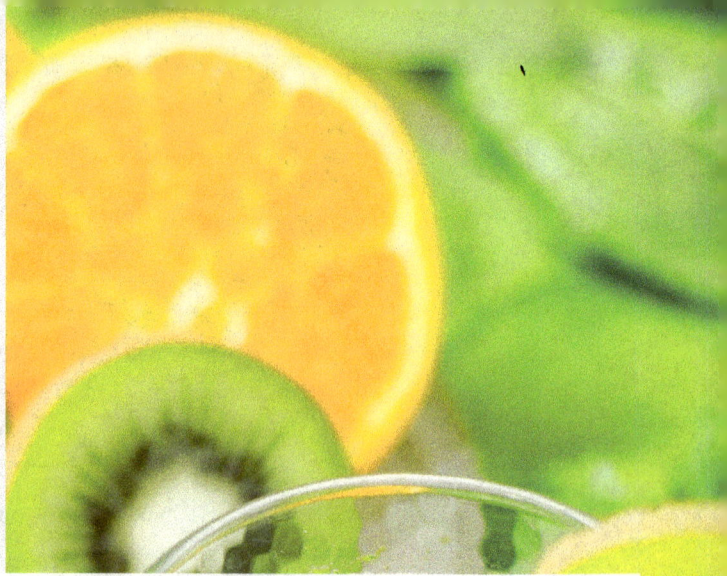

ARE SMOOTHIES HELPFUL IN THE WEIGHTLOSS?

Smoothies are the best option that can be helpful in your weight loss. Consuming an accurate smoothie with a proper lifestyle immensely reduces the weight. All you need is to create your perfect recipe that should be nutrient-dense with low caloric content.
Various kinds of weight loss smoothies have been introduced that provide adequate carbohydrates, proteins and fats while keeping the calories minimum.

The specific ingredients that are considered in the weight loss smoothie plan include chia seeds, flax seeds, avocados, nut butter and spinach. These ingredients create a feeling of fullness and help to lose weight. As per recent studies, it has also been proved that replacing a regular meal with any liquid form especially fruit/vegetable smoothie is beneficial to meltdown a few pounds.

BEAUTY BENEFITS OF SMOOTHIES

Clear skin and beauty glam is just a blender away!

All you need is a blender, some fruits or vegetables and a smoothie base. Blend them well and get clear glowy skin with mind-blowing results.

Smoothies contribute to the proper skin hydration with their anti-oxidant effect that makes you even younger and keeping the wrinkles away.

For this reason, researchers have developed a collagen-rich smoothie that helps you replenish the natural collagen supply of your body. It not only enhances the quality of the skin but also hair, nails, bones and joints.

Raspberry smoothies and banana smoothies are considered helpful in the beauty benefits of skin. Moreover, papaya smoothie is a power fruit that helps clearing the skin pores as it.

contains essential vitamins. In addition to this, kale smoothie and coconut smoothie are for glowing and repairing skin.

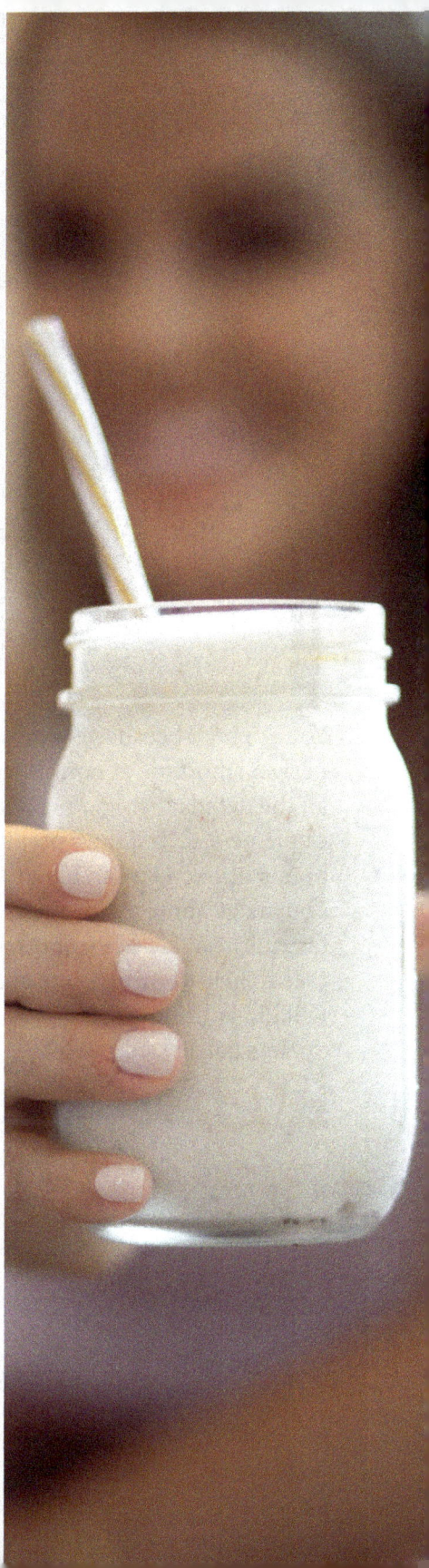

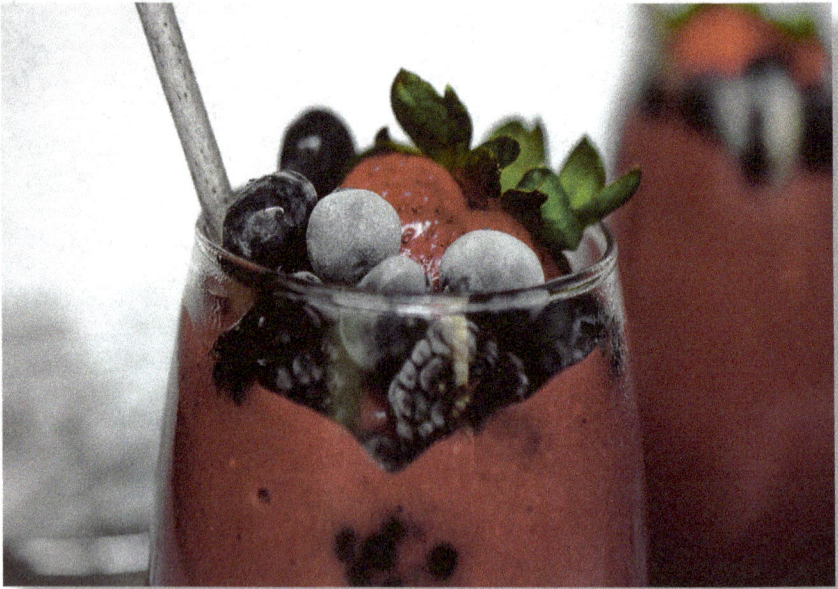

You are here because you are a smoothie lover and want to make a perfect smoothie at home. Well, ladies and gentlemen, you will get all the details that you need to know, from selecting the right tools to implement techniques, preparation guidelines, storage ideas, and some bonus tips so you can blend the perfect smoothie.

You are at home and want to make something delicious and nutritious, faster. The answer is smoothie; not only it will give you enough nutrients to help your immune system, brig flavour to your life and also it will kill your boredom.

So, let's get started.

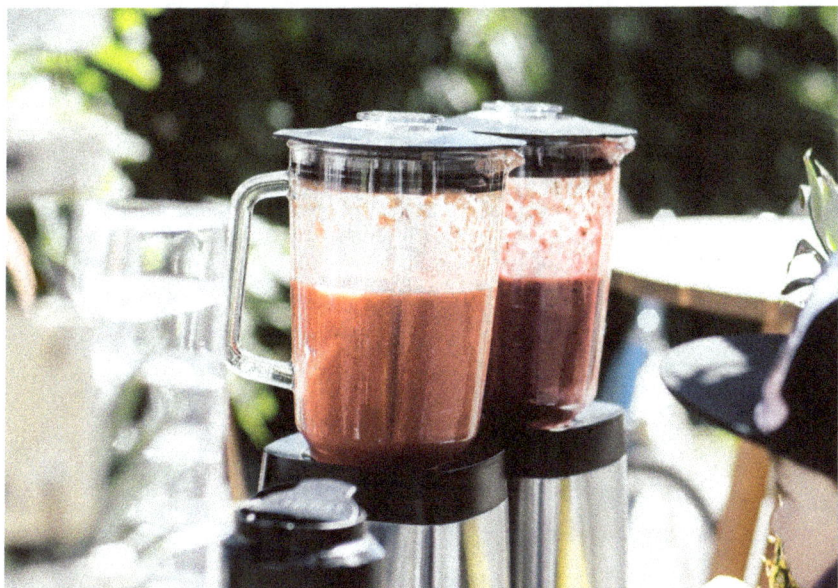

THE RIGHT KITCHEN TOOLS

To make a good smoothie, the first and foremost thing to do is to get the right kitchen tools. As you may already know that there is no better tool or equipment than a "Blender" to make a great smoothie.

This smart piece of appliance machinery was invented in 1922 by Stephen J. Poplawski. Poplawski wanted to create something that can mix his fruits and vegetables into a go-to drink form and so he designed a blender by simply placing a spinning blade at the base of the glass container.

By the time of 1935, Frederick Osius and Fred Waring made major improvements on the fundamental design and then marketed it with the famous name of "Waring Blender." What happened next in the future was just history.

Talking about the structure and dimensions of a blender, it is made of metal, plastic, or more common glass material on top that is fitted with a stainless-steel blade at the base. Below the blades is the motor and chip integrated with the control panel that lets you control the speed of the rotary blades. It blends, chops, whips, and liquefies any crushable material you put in it. You can put something that is easily crushable, which means soft fruits, vegetables, and dry fruits. It is advised not to

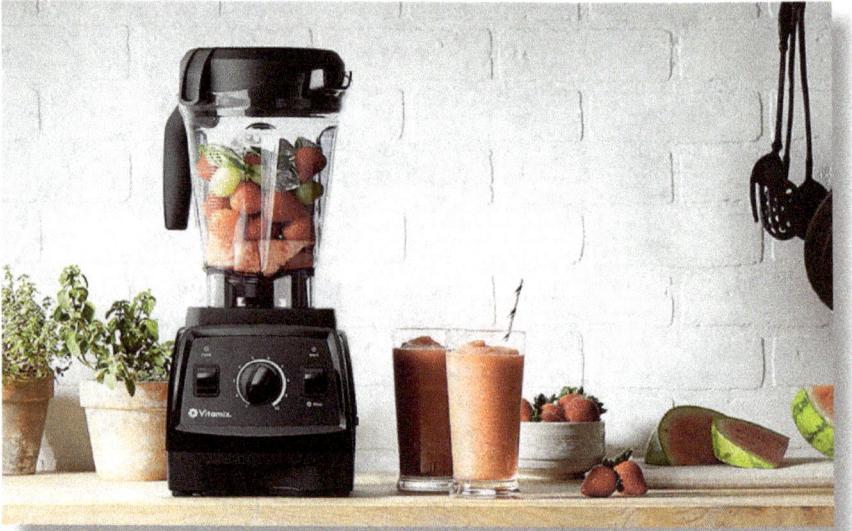

put something that is too hard so it doesn't harm the glass or mess up the blades.

Blender containers usually come in two distinct sizes: thirty-two ounces and forty ounces. If you are going to make smoothies for more than two or three people, choose a big-sized one.

Blender motors come in a variety of sizes. Those with 290-watt motors are good for most mixing operations, but not as good with smoothies. Some with 330 to 400 watts are considered to be professional and very good at crushing ice, a very important factor in creating excellent smoothies.

Blenders can be found in a variety of blade speed options, ranging from two-speed (high and low) to five and ten speeds. Variable-speed models offer many options, such as the ability to blend and whip.

CHOOSING A BLENDER

There are a variety of blender models on the market, and simply choosing a model randomly, or going with someone else's recommendations doesn't make much sense, because everyone has diverse needs and budgets.

This is where most people get really confused, so we have decided to take the challenge and make it as simple and easy as possible for you to choose a good blender that will last you for a long.

Just ask yourself what you would like to do with your blender.

That's why the first thing you need to do is to find a blender that you can be happy with for the long term. So, there are 4 main types of blenders that you should know about.

Each type has different goals and needs;

The main four types are: Hand Blenders, Traditional Countertop Blenders, Personal Bullet Blenders, and Top High-Performance Blenders.

1. Hand / Immersion Blenders

These are hand-held combinations, which often come with a variety of additives. This makes them more versatile and they can do every-thing from making soups and smoothies to marinades and even thick mayonnaise.

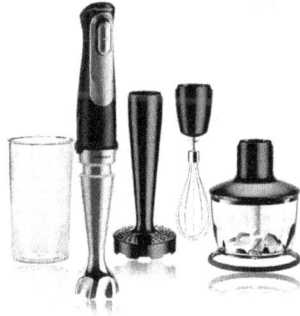

One of the great advantages of a hand blender is its compact size. If you have a small kitchen, this type of blender is the only one that does not take a huge space.

2. Countertop Blenders

As you might have got the idea from
the name, this type of blender is more
likely to stay on your kitchen counter.

They are much stronger than hand
blends but most of such models will
not be able to cope with the wide range
of smoothie ingredients as of bullet
blenders or high-performance master
chef style of smoothie blends.

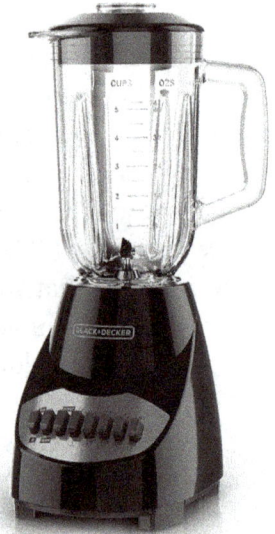

3. Personal Bullet Blenders

This type of blender is great for making one or two servings of smoothies
(depending on the model).

They are usually slightly smaller than
traditional jug-shaped blenders and
have a 9mm bullet-shaped mixing
glass cup that can be removed.

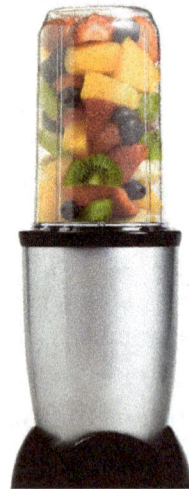

4. High-Performance Blenders

Simply put, this type of blender is the most powerful you can buy and is a Guru in dealing with the most challenging smoothie ingredients easily. The result - your smoothies will have a smooth and creamy texture that is a hallmark of that MasterChef type of blend.

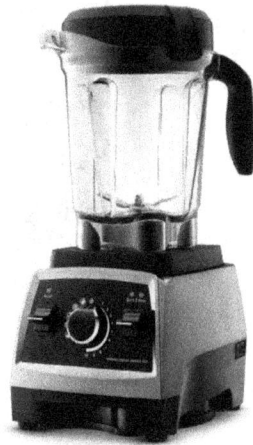

Blendtec and Vitamix are some well-known blender names in this category, but there are also a few other blenders that have done a really good job, and it is up to you to buy the right one wisely.

Some factors that you must put into consideration before selecting any blender after choosing your category are to check the brand name and its history, price, durability, warranty, and by reading some reviews on the product, the decision making will become easy for you.

PREPARATION TIPS

Here are three methods or tips to prepare for your tasty smoothie before it is time to put the goodies in the blender's jug and rev up the blades.

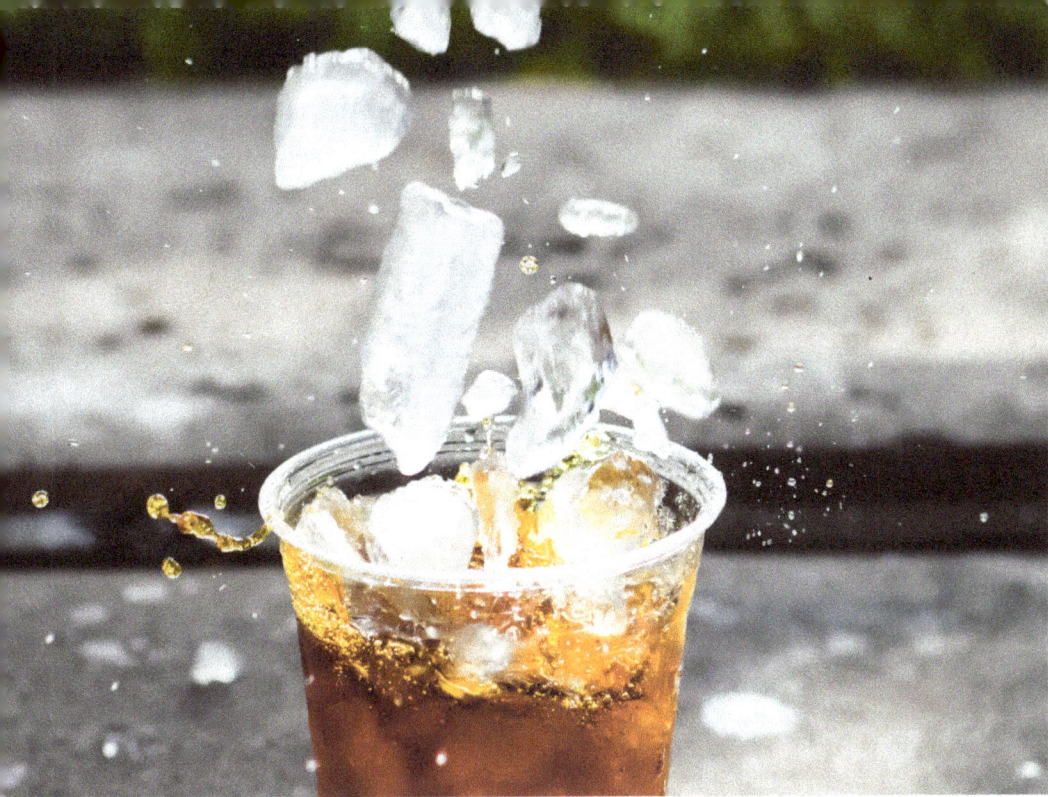

Tip 1: Ice cube tray method

The best way to make deliciously thick and cold smoothies ahead of time; because you can cherish the smoothie right away by simply crushing the ice cubes in your new blender.

What to do:

Once you have made your smoothies, pour them into an ice cube tray so that every "cube" space is evenly filled. For this, silicone trays are a good option as they are easily removable.

Place your ice tray in the deep freezer overnight, or you can make the material for up to a whole month.

When you are ready to get your favorite smoothie, put smoothie frozen cubes in a large glass-covered glass and transfer them to the refrigerator for about an hour. After that, give the glass a nice shake and that thick smoothie treat will be ready to consume!

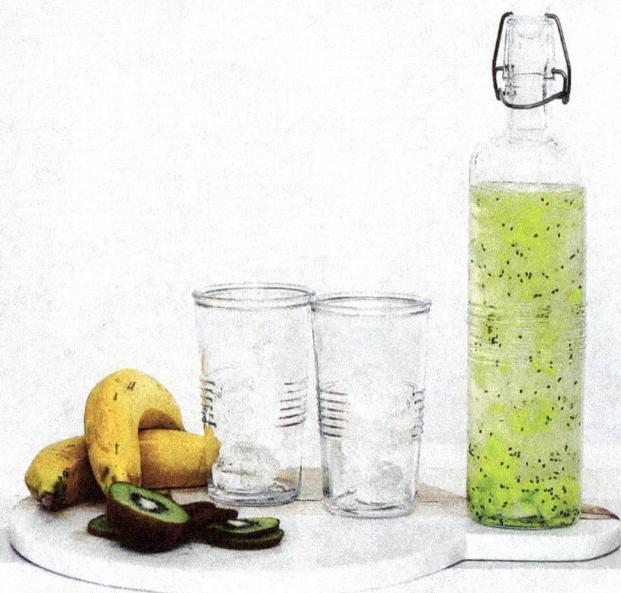

Tip 2: The glass jar technique

After you have made your smoothies to use for later on, simply buy a couple of mason jars and store the stuff in them.
You can store smoothies in that jar for as long as one month in the freezer and can simply consume them later on. Just take out the mason jar from the freezer a couple of hours before consuming or just take the frozen smoothie out at night and in the morning your smoothie breakfast will be ready

Tip 3: Wash your blender technique

Washing a dirty blender (and safely making sure the blades are clean) is both time-consuming and difficult. Just fill your dirty blender about halfway with water, add some dish soap, and turn the blender back on.
 Then all you have to do is rinse away those bubbles and you're ready to make your next smoothie.

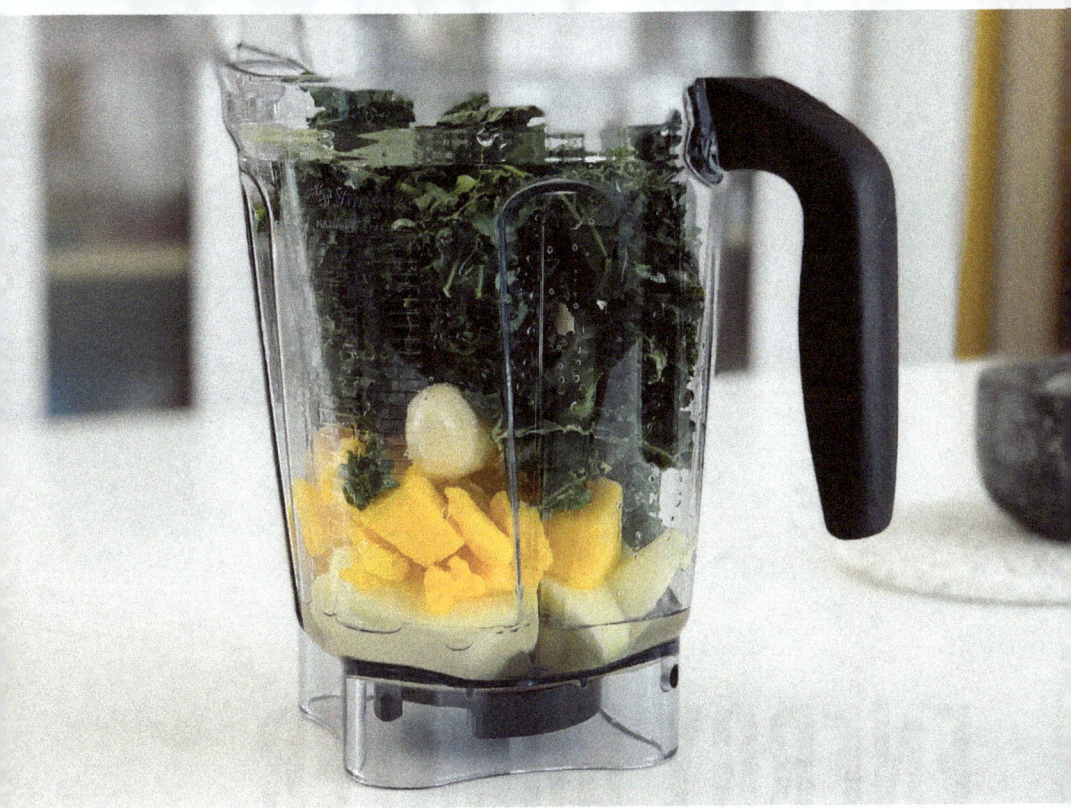

Some bonus tips to create better smoothies

- Try to read and research about different blends and trying out new taste combinations, trust me, it will never get boring this way.
- Buy a good quality blender, just don't fall for a cheap one. You may have to pay a little higher for a quality one but it will last you a lifetime and will make better blends.
- Try and make smoothies for at least a whole week and store them to consume quickly.
- Buy one with a removable glass top so you can clean it easily.

ENERGY BOOSTER SMOOTHIES

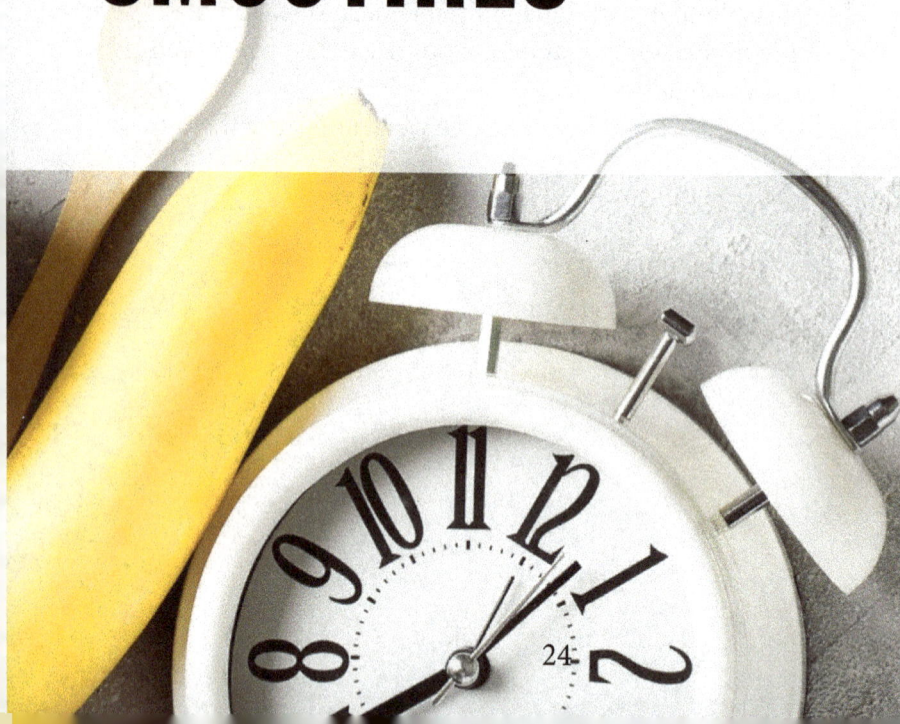

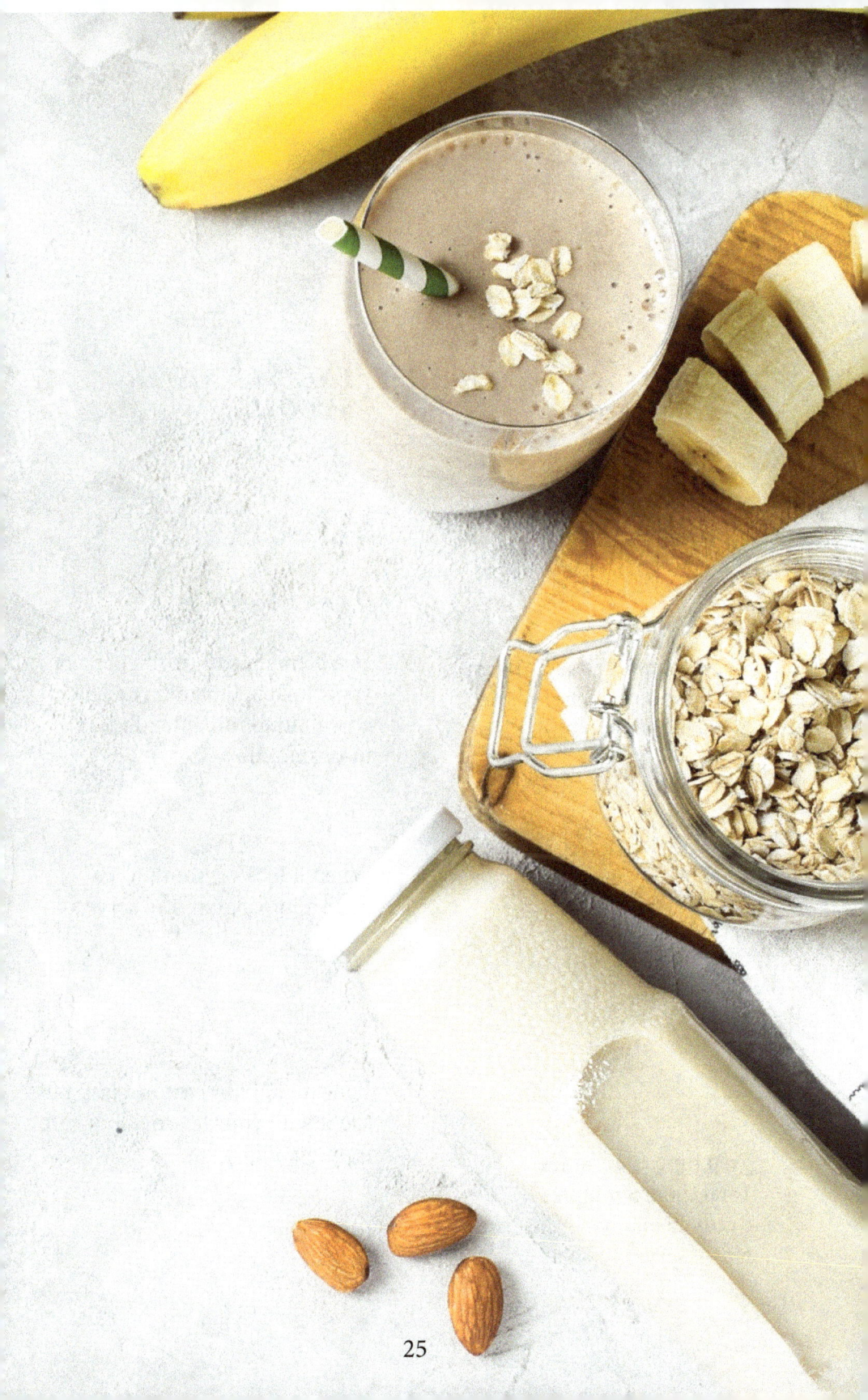

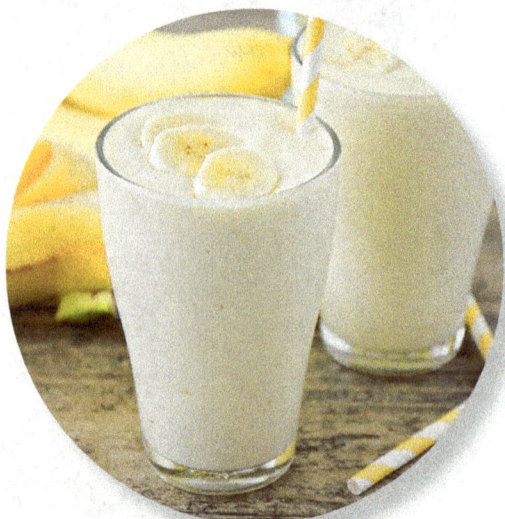

BANANA ENERGY SMOOTHIE

ENERGY BOOSTER SMOOTHIE

INGREDIENTS

- ½ cup almond milk
- ¾ cup banana cream Yogurt
- 2 tablespoons Delight French vanilla creamer
- 2 frozen bananas

INSTRUCTIONS

01 In a blender, add frozen bananas, yogurt, Delight vanilla creamer, and almond milk blend them until smooth.

02 When it looks smooth, then pour it into a glass and serve.

03 Pour the mixture into a glass and top it with your favorite low-carb topping. Enjoy!

PREP TIME & SERVING

Prep time: 5 minutes
Total time: 5 minutes
Ready in about: 5 mins
No. of serve: 1

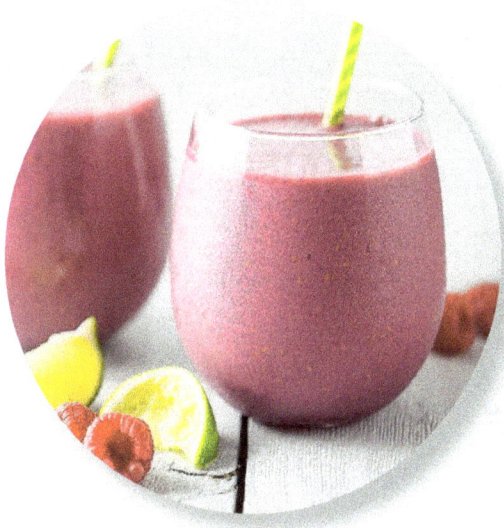

RASPBERRY LIME SMOOTHIE

ENERGY BOOSTER SMOOTHIE

INGREDIENTS

- 2 cups limeade
- 1 cup key lime pie Yogurt
- 2 cups frozen raspberries

INSTRUCTIONS

01 In a blender, add limeade, yogurt, and raspberries blend for 2 minutes.

02 When it looks smooth, then pour it into a glass. Serve right away

PREP TIME & SERVING

Prep time: 6 minutes
Total time: 6 minutes
Ready in about: 6 mins
No. of serve: 1

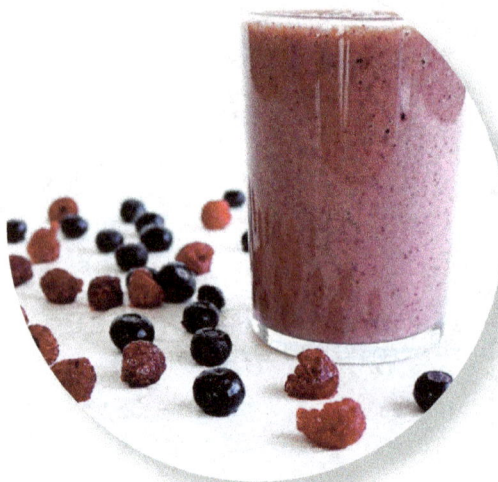

BERRY ENERGY BOOST SMOOTHIE

ENERGY BOOSTER SMOOTHIE

INGREDIENTS

- 1 cup frozen strawberries
- 1 cup raspberries
- 1 cup milk
- 3 tablespoons sugar
- 1 cup ice

INSTRUCTIONS

01 Thoroughly mix all ingredients in a high-speed blender and blend them for a minute.

02 When it looks smooth, then pour it into a glass and serve. Enjoy!

PREP TIME & SERVING

Prep time: 3 minutes
Total time: 5 minutes
Ready in about: 5 mins
No. of serve: 1

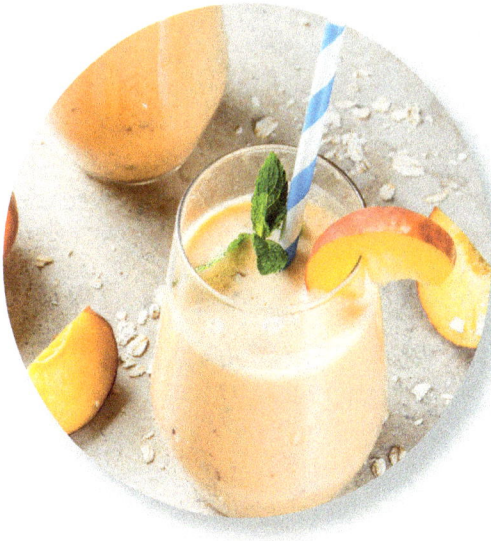

PEACHES & CREAM SMOOTHIE

ENERGY BOOSTER SMOOTHIE

INGREDIENTS

- 2 cups frozen peaches
- ½ cup heavy cream
- ½ cup milk
- 1 tablespoon honey
- A splash of vanilla extract
- Pinch of cinnamon

PREP TIME & SERVING

Prep time: 5 minutes
Total time: 5 minutes
Ready in about: 5 mins
No. of serve: 1

INSTRUCTIONS

01 Grab a strong blender add frozen peaches with cream and milk.

02 Add the rest ingredients in the end and blend until it gives a smooth texture.

03 When the required texture is produced, then pour it into a glass and serve.

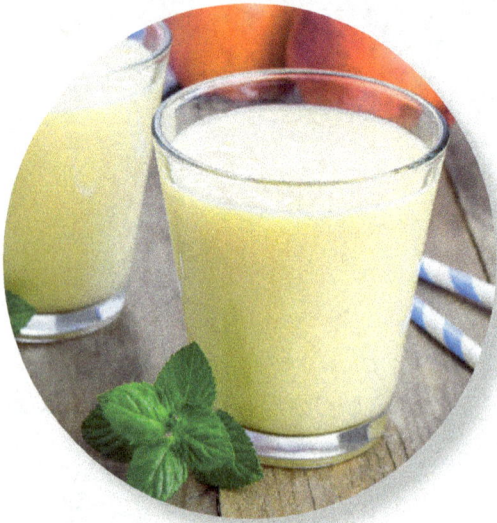

APPLE ENERGY BOSST SMOOTHIE

ENERGY BOOSTER SMOOTHIE

INGREDIENTS

- Handful of watercress
- 1 peach
- ¼ avocado
- Handful fresh mint
- ¼ cup apple juice
- 1 cup water

INSTRUCTIONS

01 Take a blender, add watercress, peach, avocado, mint, apple juice, and water blend them until smooth.

02 When it looks smooth, then pour it into a glass. Serve.

PREP TIME & SERVING

Prep time: 5 minutes
Total time: 5 minutes
Ready in about: 5 mins
No. of serve: 1

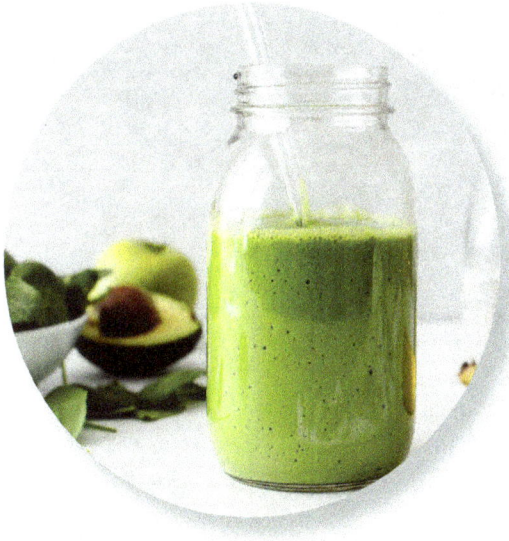

KALE PINEAPPLE ENERGY SMOOTHIE

ENERGY BOOSTER SMOOTHIE

INGREDIENTS

- ¼ cup frozen pineapple
- 1 cup kale
- 1 tablespoon coconut oil
- ½ avocado
- 1 cup coconut water
- 1 teaspoon matcha green tea (optional)

INSTRUCTIONS

01 Add frozen pineapple, kale, and avocado with coconut water.

02 Also, add the coconut oil and blend until it comes in a smooth form.

03 When the required consistency looks, then pour it into a glass and serve.

PREP TIME & SERVING

Prep time: 5 minutes
Total time: 10 minutes
Ready in about: 10 mins
No. of serve: 1

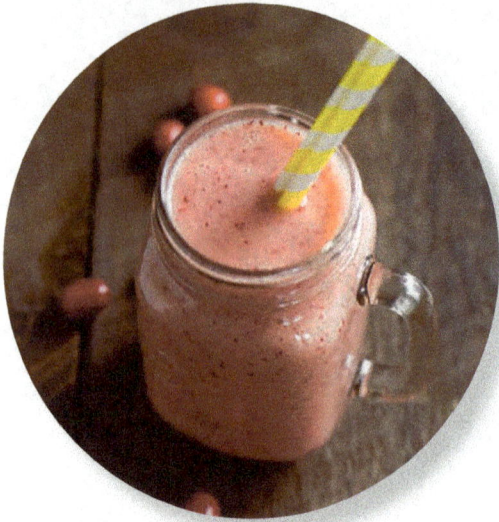

SUPER ENERGY CRANBERRY APPLE

ENERGY BOOSTER SMOOTHIE

INGREDIENTS

- 1 apple peeled
- 1 cup frozen or fresh cranberries
- ½ frozen banana
- 1 teaspoon maple syrup (optional)
- ½ cup coconut milk
- 1 teaspoon chia seeds
- 1 teaspoon lemon juice
- Pinch of ground cinnamon

INSTRUCTIONS

01 Thoroughly mix all ingredients at a high-speed and blend them for a minute.

02 When it looks smooth, then pour it into a glass and serve.

PREP TIME & SERVING

Prep time: 5 minutes
Total time: 5 minutes
Ready in about: 5 mins
No. of serve: 2

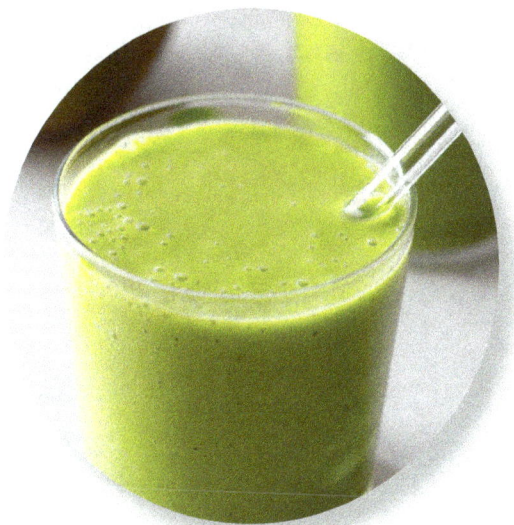

CITRUS ENERGY BOOST SMOOTHIE

ENERGY BOOSTER SMOOTHIE

INGREDIENTS

- 2 cups spinach or kale
- 1 cup water
- 2 oranges
- 1 cup frozen chopped pineapple
- 1 cup chopped mango
- 2 tablespoons chia seeds

INSTRUCTIONS

01 Take a blender, add spinach and oranges, and water blend until smooth.

02 Also, add mango, pineapple, and chia seeds and blend again.

03 When it looks smooth, then pour it into a glass and serve

PREP TIME & SERVING

Prep time: 5 minutes
Total time: 5 minutes
Ready in about: 5 mins
No. of serve: 1

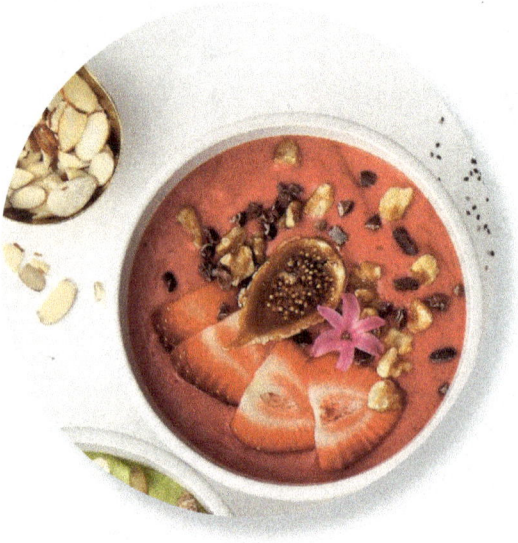

RED BERRY SMOOTHIE BOWL

ENERGY BOOSTER SMOOTHIE

INGREDIENTS

- 1 cup frozen raspberries
- 1 cup frozen strawberries
- 1 cup chopped romaine stems
- 1 apple, chopped
- 1 frozen banana
- ½ cup plain Yogurt
- 1 tsp honey

INSTRUCTIONS

01 Grab a strong blender add frozen raspberries, strawberries, apple, banana, yogurt, romaine stems, and honey blend until smooth.

02 When it looks smooth, then pour into 2 bowls. Serve.

PREP TIME & SERVING

Prep time: 10 minutes
Total time: 10 minutes
Ready in about: 10 mins
No. of serve: 2

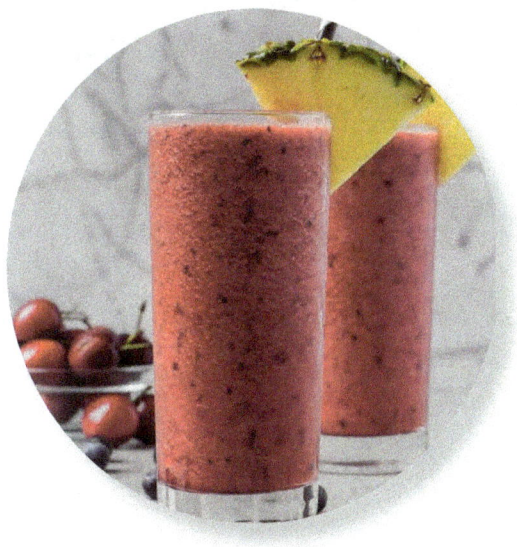

CHERRY PINEAPPLE SMOOTHIE

ENERGY BOOSTER SMOOTHIE

INGREDIENTS

- 1 frozen banana
- 1 cup fresh cherries
- 1 cup pineapple chopped
- ½ cup almond milk
- 1 tablespoon chia seeds
- 3 cups of ice
- 1 tablespoon maple syrup (optional)

PREP TIME & SERVING

Prep time: 5 minutes
Total time: 5 minutes
Ready in about: 5 mins
No. of serve: 2

INSTRUCTIONS

01 Take a blender to add frozen banana, fresh cherries, pineapple, and chia seeds with almond milk.

02 Also, add the rest ingredients and blend for a few minutes.

03 When it looks smooth, then pour it into glasses. Serve right away.

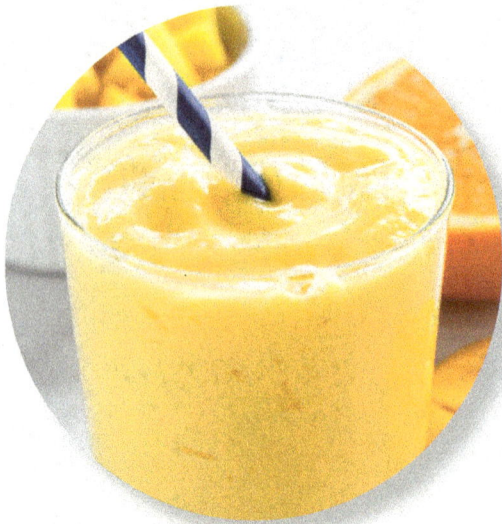

MANGO ENERGY BOOST SMOOTHIE

ENERGY BOOSTER SMOOTHIE

INGREDIENTS

- ½ cup almond milk
- 2 cups baby spinach
- 1 frozen banana
- ¾ cup frozen mango
- Half lemon juice
- 1 tablespoon chia seeds
- 1 tablespoon almond butter (optional)

INSTRUCTIONS

01 Grab a strong blender add spinach, frozen banana, frozen mango, chia seeds, and almond milk, and blend them for a couple of minutes.

02 When the required texture is produced, then pour it into glasses. Enjoy!

PREP TIME & SERVING

Prep time: 5 minutes
Total time: 5 minutes
Ready in about: 5 mins
No. of serve: 2

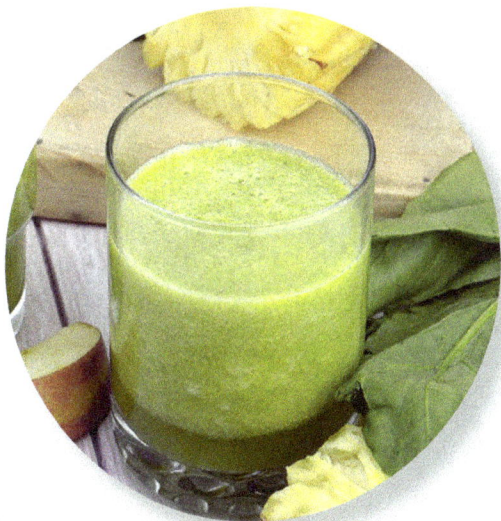

CELERY SPINACH ENERGY BOOSTING SMOOTHIE

ENERGY BOOSTER SMOOTHIE

INGREDIENTS

- 1 stalk celery
- 2 cup fresh spinach
- 2 fresh pineapple slices
- 2 cups almond milk

PREP TIME & SERVING

Prep time: 3 minutes
Total time: 5 minutes
Ready in about: 5 mins
No. of serve: 2

INSTRUCTIONS

01 Wash the spinach and celery and roughly chopped.

02 Take a blender, add chopped celery, spinach, and pineapple with almond milk, and blend until smooth.

03 When the required consistency looks, then pour it into glasses and serve.

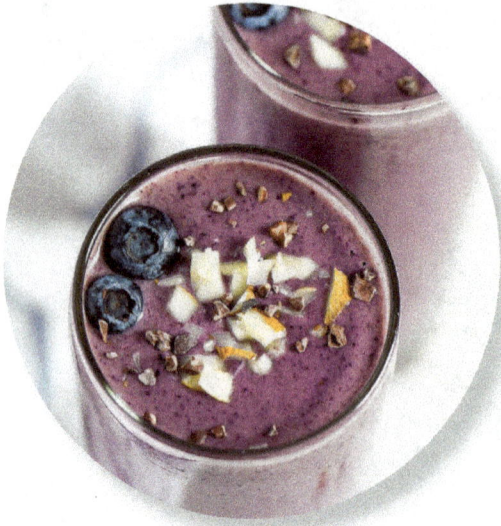

BLUEBERRY ENEGY BOOSTING SMOOTHIE

ENERGY BOOSTER SMOOTHIE

INGREDIENTS

- 2/3 cups frozen blueber-ries
- ½ cup milk
- 1/3 cup vanilla Greek Yogurt
- 1 banana
- 1 tablespoon rolled oats
- Pinch of cinnamon

PREP TIME & SERVING

Prep time: 7 minutes
Total time: 10 minutes
Ready in about: 10 mins
No. of serve: 1

INSTRUCTIONS

01 Grab a high-speed blender and blend all these ingredients.

02 Blend them well until it turns in a smooth form.

03 When the required consistency looks, then pour into a glass and enjoy.

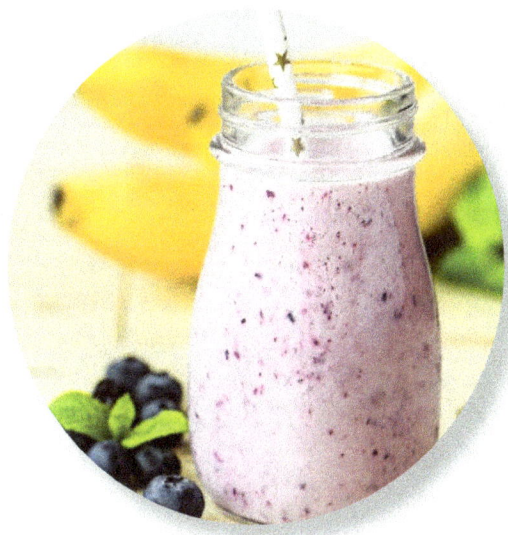

ENERGY BOOSTING BERRY BANANA SMOOTHIE

ENERGY BOOSTER SMOOTHIE

INGREDIENTS

- 1 cup frozen strawberries
- ¼ cup dates
- 3 tablespoons beaming protein blend with greens
- 3 tablespoon hemp seeds
- 1 cup almond milk
- 1 banana

INSTRUCTIONS

01 Add frozen strawberries, dates, banana, and almond milk.

02 Also, add the rest ingredients to a blender and blend them until smooth.

03 When the required consistency looks, then pour it into a glass. Serve

PREP TIME & SERVING

Prep time: 5 minutes
Total time: 5 minutes
Ready in about: 5 mins
No. of serve: 1

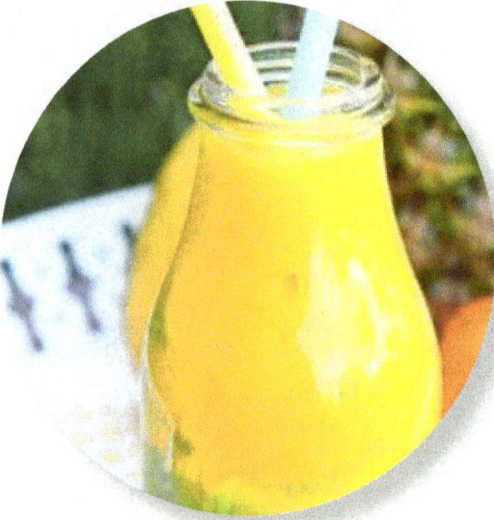

SUNBURST ENERGY SMOOTHIE

ENERGY BOOSTER SMOOTHIE

INGREDIENTS

- ¾ cup frozen pineapple
- ¾ cup frozen mango
- ¾ cup orange juice
- 1 banana
- 1 tbsp chia seeds

INSTRUCTIONS

01 Mix all ingredients in a high-speed blender and blend them for a minute.

02 When it looks smooth, then pour it into glasses, and serve.

PREP TIME & SERVING

Prep time: 5 minutes
Total time: 5 minutes
Ready in about: 5 mins
No. of serve: 4

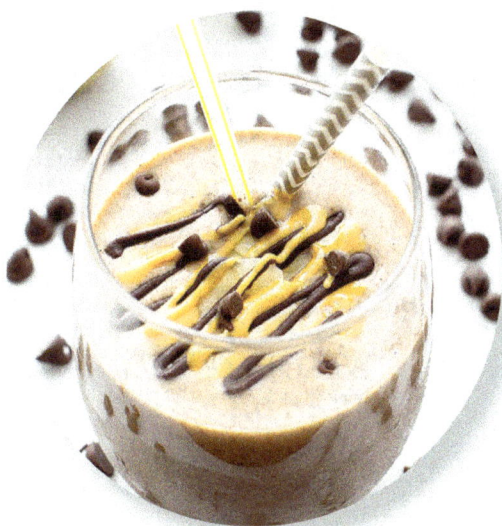

CHOCOLATE PEANUT BUTTER SMOOTHIE

ENERGY BOOSTER SMOOTHIE

INGREDIENTS

- 1 frozen banana
- 2 tablespoon peanut butter powder
- 1 tablespoon cacao powder
- 1 tablespoon maca powder
- 1 cup almond milk

INSTRUCTIONS

01 Add peanut butter powder, banana, maca powder, cacao powder, and almond milk in a blender. Blend until smooth.

02 When it looks smooth, then pour it into a glass and serve.

PREP TIME & SERVING

Prep time: 5 minutes
Total time: 5 minutes
Ready in about: 5 mins
No. of serve: 1

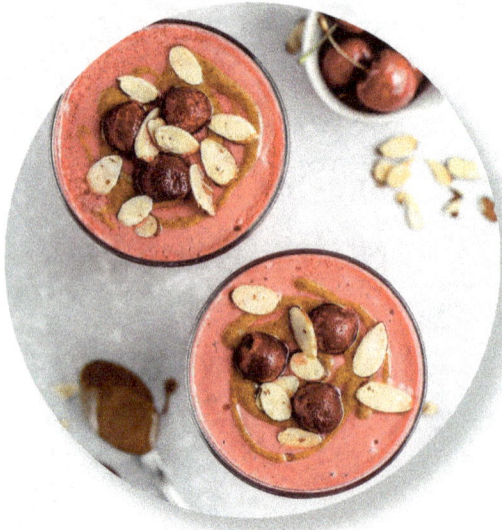

SWEET CHERRY ALMOND SMOOTHIE

ENERGY BOOSTER SMOOTHIE

INGREDIENTS

- 1 ½ cups frozen cherries
- 1 cup almond milk
- 1 scoop protein powder
- 1 banana
- 3 ice cubes

INSTRUCTIONS

01 Take a blender to add frozen cherries, protein powder, and banana with almond milk blend until smooth and creamy.

02 When the required consistency looks then pour into a glass and enjoy.

PREP TIME & SERVING

Prep time: 5 minutes
Total time: 5 minutes
Ready in about: 5 mins
No. of serve: 1

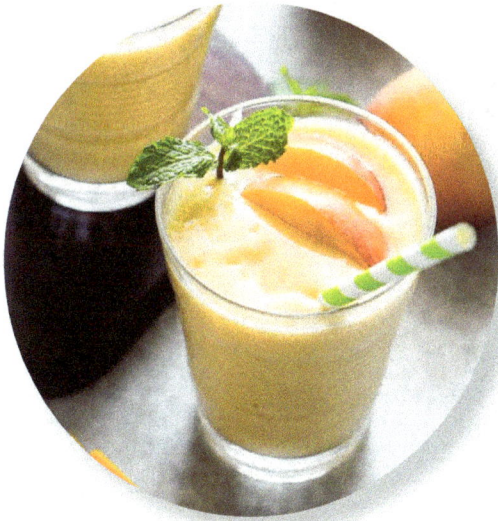

PEACHY MANGO SMOOTHIE

ENERGY BOOSTER SMOOTHIE

INGREDIENTS

- 1 cup peaches
- 1 cup mangoes
- 1 banana
- 1 cup orange juice
- ¼ teaspoon turmeric
- ¼ teaspoon ginger

INSTRUCTIONS

01 Take a high-speed blender and add peaches, mangoes, banana, turmeric, and ginger with orange juice and blend them for a few minutes.

02 When it looks smooth, then pour it into a glass and serve.

PREP TIME & SERVING

Prep time: 5 minutes
Total time: 5 minutes
Ready in about: 5 mins
No. of serve: 1

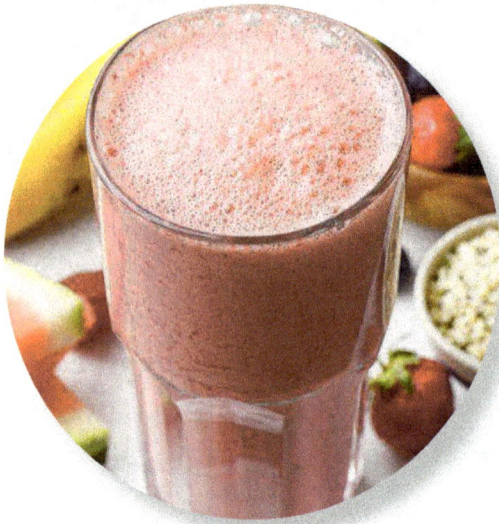

SUPER ENERGY SMOOTHIE

ENERGY BOOSTER SMOOTHIE

INGREDIENTS

- 4 cups pineapple
- 4 cups watermelon
- 8 cups coconut water
- 1 bunch spinach
- 1-2 cups blueberries
- 2 green apples

INSTRUCTIONS

01 Take a high-speed blender, add watermelon, pineapple, blueberries, apples, and spinach with coconut water blend them for a minute.

02 When it looks smooth, then pour it into glasses. Serve immediately.

PREP TIME & SERVING

Prep time: 5 minutes
Total time: 5 minutes
Ready in about: 5 mins
No. of serve: 4

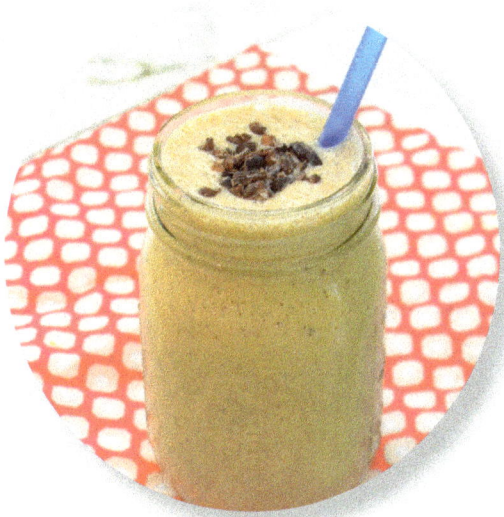

HIGH PROTEIN SUPER ENERGY SMOOTHIE

ENERGY BOOSTER SMOOTHIE

INGREDIENTS

- 2 tablespoons almond butter
- 1 tablespoon rolled oats
- 1 tablespoon honey
- 1 scoop protein powder
- 1 banana
- ¾ tablespoon maca powder
- ¾ tablespoon cocoa nibs
- 1.5 cups unsweetened almond milk
- A handful of ice cubes

INSTRUCTIONS

01 Use a high-speed blender and blend them until smooth.

02 When it looks smooth, then pour it into glasses. Serve right away.

PREP TIME & SERVING

Prep time: 5 minutes
Total time: 5 minutes
Ready in about: 5 mins
No. of serve: 2

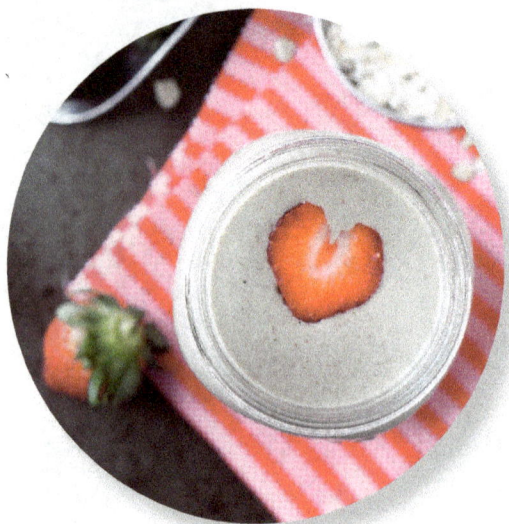

ENERGY BOOSTING OATMEAL BERRY SMOOTHIE

ENERGY BOOSTER SMOOTHIE

INGREDIENTS

- 1 frozen banana
- 1 cup almond milk
- 1 cup frozen berries
- 1 cup rolled oats
- 1 tablespoon honey
- 1 tablespoon chia seeds

PREP TIME & SERVING

Prep time: 5 minutes
Total time: 5 minutes
Ready in about: 5 mins
No. of serve: 2

INSTRUCTIONS

01 In a blender, add frozen berries, bananas, and oats with almond milk.

02 Also, add the rest ingredients and blend them until very smooth.

03 When it looks smooth, then pour it into glasses and serve.

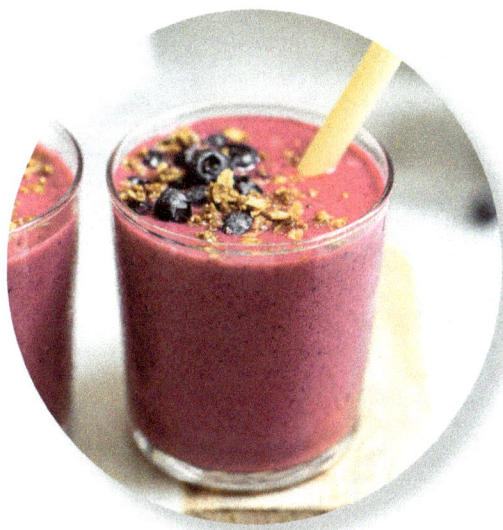

BEET BERRY APPLE CHIA SMOOTHIE

*ENERGY BOOSTER
SMOOTHIE*

INGREDIENTS

- 2 cups frozen blueberries
- 1 cup unsweetened apple juice
- 1 cup full-fat coconut milk
- 1 tablespoon chia seeds
- 1/8 teaspoon ground cinnamon
- 3 small beets

PREP TIME & SERVING

Prep time: 5 minutes
Total time: 5 minutes
Ready in about: 5 mins
No. of serve: 2

INSTRUCTIONS

01 Take a high-powered blender and add blueberries, beets, and coconut milk.

02 Also, add apple juice, chia seeds, and cinnamon, blend them until very smooth and creamy.

03 When it looks smooth, then pour it into glasses. Serve and enjoy!

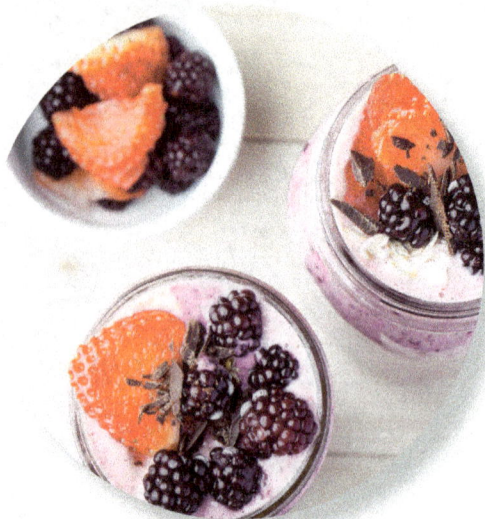

BLACKBERRY ENERGY BOOSTER SMOOTHIE

ENERGY BOOSTER SMOOTHIE

INGREDIENTS

- 1cup frozen blackberries
- ½ cup frozen raspberries
- 1 banana
- ½ avocado
- 2 cups baby spinach
- 1/3 cup fresh mint
- ½ cup water
- 1/3 cup almonds
- 4 ice cubes

INSTRUCTIONS

01 Mix all ingredients in a high-speed blender and blend at high speed for 1 minute.

02 When it looks smooth, then pour it into glasses. Serve

PREP TIME & SERVING

Prep time: 5 minutes
Total time: 5 minutes
Ready in about: 5 mins
No. of serve: 1

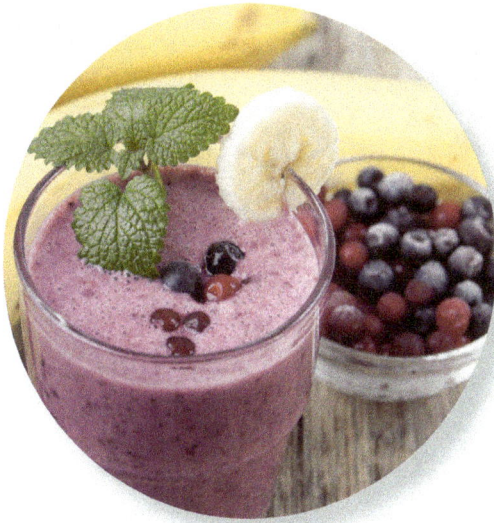

CRANBERRY ENERGY BOOSTING SMOOTHIE

ENERGY BOOSTER SMOOTHIE

INGREDIENTS

- 1 frozen banana
- 1 cup baby spinach
- ½ cup cranberries
- ½ cup blueberries
- 2 cups cold water
- 2 teaspoons Camu Camu powder
- 2 teaspoon gelatinized maca powder
- I tablespoon hemp seeds
- 3 tablespoons ground flax-seeds
- 5 Medjool dates
- 1 teaspoon vanilla extract
- Pinch of sea salt
- 1 ½ cups ice

PREP TIME & SERVING

Prep time: 5 minutes
Total time: 5 minutes
Ready in about: 5 mins
No. of serve: 2

INSTRUCTIONS

01 Take a high-speed blender and add frozen banana, cranberries, blueberries, and spinach with a cold water blend.

02 Also, add the rest ingredients and blend them again when it looks smooth and creamy.

03 Then pour it into two glasses and serve.

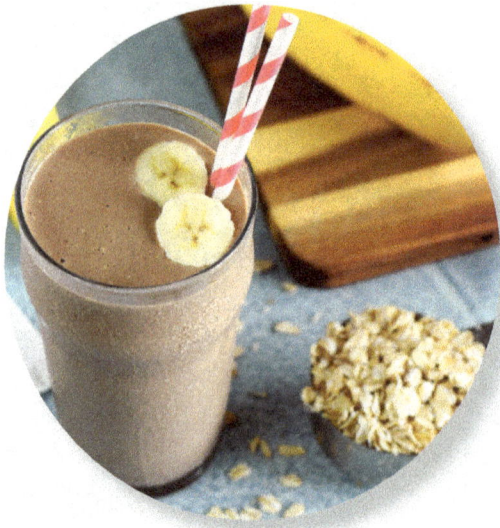

CREAMY CHOCOLATE OATMEAL SMOOTHIE

ENERGY BOOSTER SMOOTHIE

INGREDIENTS

- 2 frozen bananas
- 2 tablespoons maca powder
- 2 tablespoons unsweetened cacao powder
- ½ teaspoon Camu Camu powder
- ¼ cup old fashioned rolled oats
- 5 pitted dates
- 1 teaspoon vanilla extract
- 1 ¾ cup coconut milk
- I cup ice

PREP TIME & SERVING

Prep time: 5 minutes
Total time: 5 minutes
Ready in about: 5 mins
No. of serve: 2

INSTRUCTIONS

01 Grab a strong blender add frozen bananas, oats, and dates with coconut milk.

02 Also, add vanilla extract, maca powder, Camu Camu powder, cacao powder, and ice blend them until it gives a smooth texture.

03 When the required texture is produced, then pour it into glasses. Serve right away.

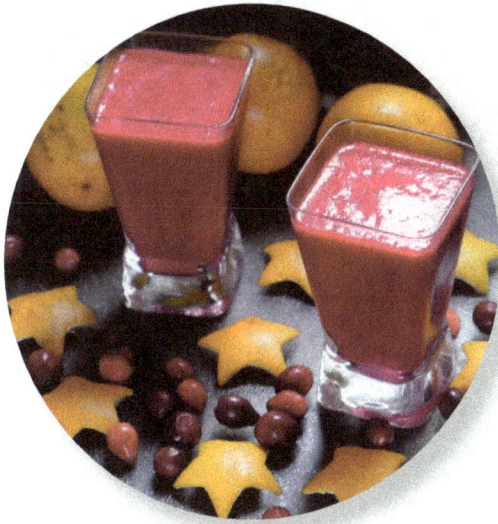

ORANGE CHERRY SMOOTHIE

ENERGY BOOSTER SMOOTHIE

INGREDIENTS

- ¼ cup cherry juice
- ¼ cup fresh orange juice
- ½ cup water
- ½ cup frozen raspberries
- 1 tablespoon beet boost powder
- 1 tablespoon goji berries
- 2 pitted dates
- ½ cup water
- 1 tablespoon tocotrienols (optional)

INSTRUCTIONS

01 Take a blender, adds all the ingredients to a blender, and blend them for a few minutes.

02 When the required consistency looks, then pour into glasses. Serve

PREP TIME & SERVING

Prep time: 5 minutes
Total time: 5 minutes
Ready in about: 5 mins
No. of serve: 2

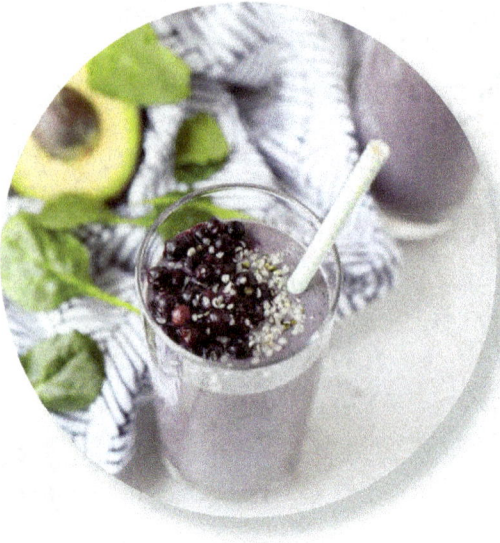

VEGAN ENERGY BOOSTING SMOOTHIE

ENERGY BOOSTER SMOOTHIE

INGREDIENTS

- 1 cup frozen blueberries
- ½ cup frozen strawberries
- ½ frozen banana
- ½ cup baby spinach
- ½ avocado
- 1/3 cup silken tofu
- ¼ cup walnuts
- 1 teaspoon hemp seeds
- 1-2 Medjool dates
- 1 cup unsweetened almond milk

INSTRUCTIONS

01 Thoroughly mix all ingredients in a high-speed blender and them for a minute.

02 When it looks smooth, then pour it into a glass and serve.

PREP TIME & SERVING

Prep time: 5 minutes
Total time: 5 minutes
Ready in about: 5 mins
No. of serve: 1

SKINNY BANANA SPLIT PROTEIN SMOOTHIE

ENERGY BOOSTER SMOOTHIE

INGREDIENTS

- ½ cup non-fat Greek yogurt
- ½ cup almond milk
- 1 tablespoon almonds
- ½ cup strawberries
- 1 banana peeled
- 2 tablespoons protein powder
- Ice cubes

PREP TIME & SERVING

Prep time: 5 minutes
Total time: 5 minutes
Ready in about: 5 mins
No. of serve: 2

INSTRUCTIONS

01 Take a high-speed blender to add Greek Yogurt, banana, strawberries, and almond with almond milk.

02 Also, add the rest ingredients and blend them again until smooth and creamy.

03 When it looks smooth, then pour it into glasses. Serve immediately.

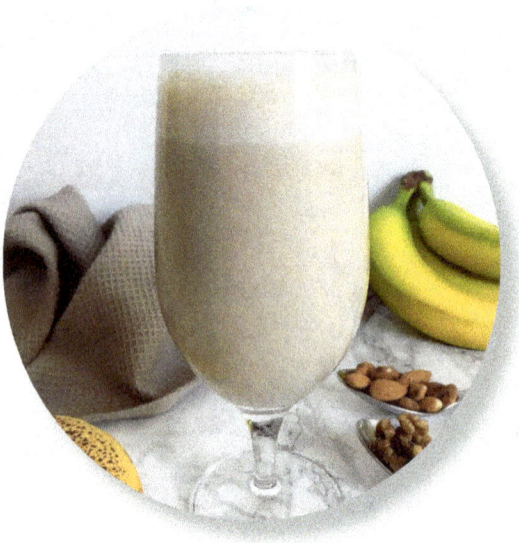

ALMOND ENERGY BOOST SMOOTHIE

ENERGY BOOSTER SMOOTHIE

INGREDIENTS

- 14 raw almonds
- 1 frozen banana
- 1 apple peeled
- 1 cup almond milk

INSTRUCTIONS

01 Add almonds, frozen banana, and apple with almond milk blend them until smooth and creamy.

02 When it looks smooth, then pour it into a glass, and serve.

PREP TIME & SERVING

Prep time: 5 minutes
Total time: 5 minutes
Ready in about: 5 mins
No. of serve: 1

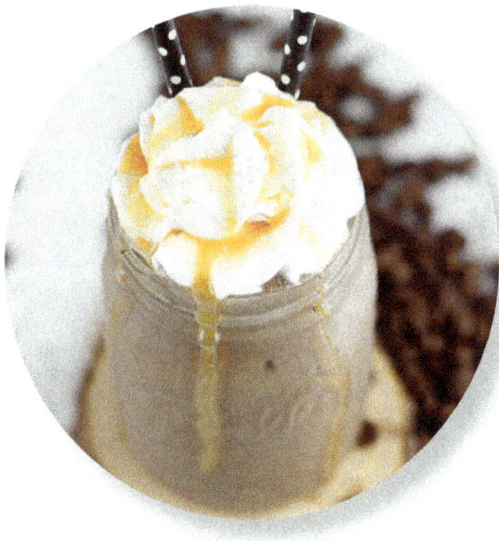

CARAMEL MOCHA SMOOTHIE

ENERGY BOOSTER SMOOTHIE

INGREDIENTS

- ½ cup cold coffee
- ½ cup unsweetened almond milk
- 1 packet sweetened cocoa powder
- 1 small frozen banana
- 1 teaspoon vanilla extract
- 3 pitted dates
- Pinch of salt
- 1 cub of ice

INSTRUCTIONS

01 Add entire ingredients in a blender, and blend for a couple of minutes or until smooth.

02 When it looks smooth, then pour it into a glass and serve.

PREP TIME & SERVING

Prep time: 5 minutes
Total time: 5 minutes
Ready in about: 5 mins
No. of serve: 1

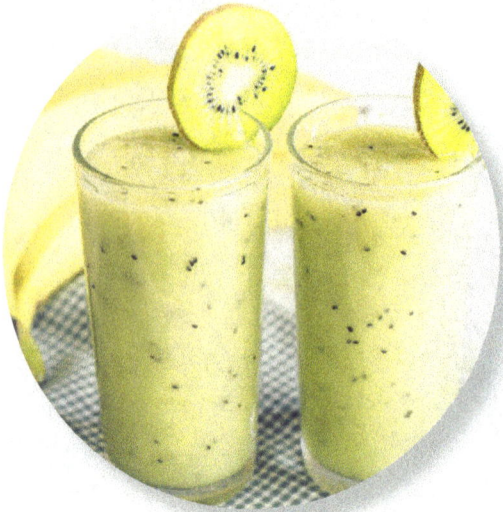

KIWI BANANA SMOOTHIE

*ENERGY BOOSTER
SMOOTHIE*

INGREDIENTS

- 2 kiwifruits peeled
- 1 banana
- ½ cup almond milk
- 1 lime juice
- 1 cup vanilla Greek Yogurt
- 1 cup ice

INSTRUCTIONS

01 Wash and peel the banana and kiwi. Take a blender, add kiwi, banana, lime juice, milk, yogurt, and ice blend them until very well.

02 When it looks smooth, then pour it into a glass, and serve.

PREP TIME & SERVING

Prep time: 5 minutes
Total time: 5 minutes
Ready in about: 5 mins
No. of serve: 2

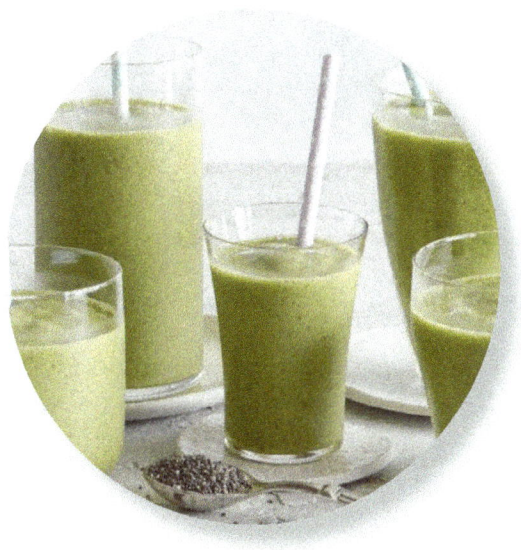

BANANA CHIA SMOOTHIE

ENERGY BOOSTER
SMOOTHIE

INGREDIENTS

- 1 ½ frozen bananas
- Handful of spinach
- 2 tablespoon peanut butter
- 1 tablespoon chia seeds
- 1 teaspoon maca powder
- 1 cup coconut water
- 1 cup cashew milk
- 2 dates
- 1 teaspoon cinnamon
- ¼ cup ice cubes

INSTRUCTIONS

01 Use a high-speed blender, and add the entire ingredients in it.

02 Blend them for a couple of minutes.

03 When it looks smooth, then pour it into a glass. Serve.

PREP TIME & SERVING

Prep time: 5 minutes
Total time: 10 minutes
Ready in about: 10 mins
No. of serve: 1

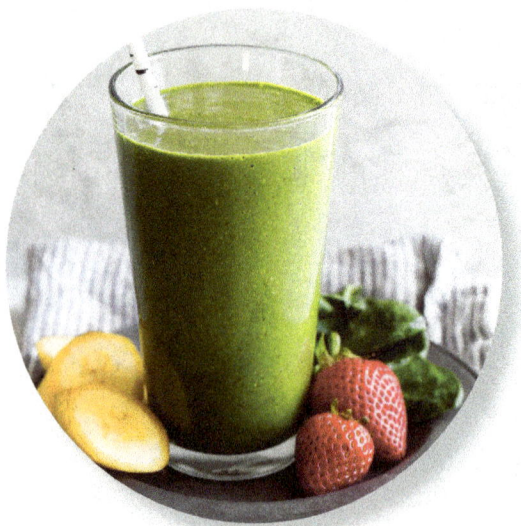

VERY BERRY ENERGY SMOOTHIE

ENERGY BOOSTER SMOOTHIE

INGREDIENTS

- ½ cup unsweetened almond milk
- 1 cup fresh spinach
- 1 banana
- ½ avocado
- 2 cups frozen blueberries
- 1 tablespoon ground flaxseed
- 1 tablespoon almond butter
- ¼ teaspoon cinnamon

PREP TIME & SERVING

Prep time: 5 minutes
Total time: 5 minutes
Ready in about: 5 mins
No. of serve: 1

INSTRUCTIONS

01 Take a strong blender, add spinach, banana, and blueberries with almond milk blend them.

02 Also, add the other ingredients and blend again.

03 When the required consistency is produced, then pour it into a glass and serve.

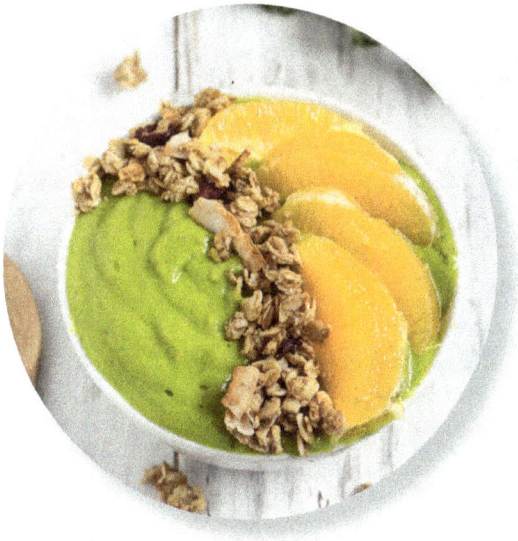

ORANGE KALE QUINOA SMOOTHIE

ENERGY BOOSTER SMOOTHIE

INGREDIENTS

- 2 oranges
- 1 orange zest
- 1 handful kale
- ¼ cup cooked quinoa
- ¼ cup almond milk
- ¼ avocado
- 1 frozen banana
- ½ teaspoon turmeric
- ¼ teaspoon cinnamon
- Orange slices for (topping)

PREP TIME & SERVING

Prep time: 10 minutes
Total time: 10 minutes
Ready in about: 10 mins
No. of serve: 2

INSTRUCTIONS

01 Grab a strong blender add oranges, kale, avocado, banana, and almond milk.

02 Also, add the other ingredients and blend them for a minute.

03 When the desired consistency is achieved, then pour it into glasses and serve.

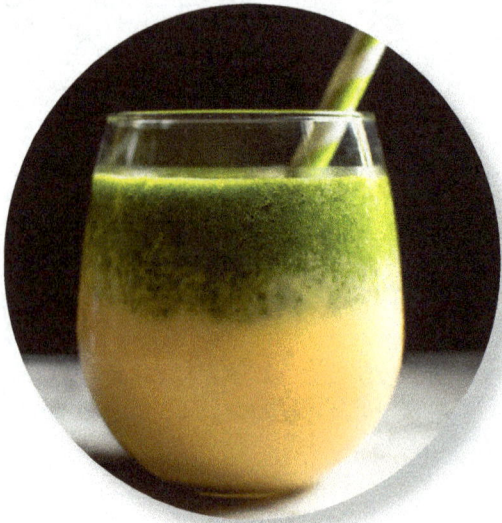

PINEAPPLE KALE ENERGY SMOOTHIE

ENERGY BOOSTER SMOOTHIE

INGREDIENTS

- ¼ cup frozen pineapple
- 1 cup kale
- 1 tablespoon coconut oil
- ½ avocado
- 1 cup coconut water
- 1 teaspoon matcha green tea (optional)
- ½ cup full-fat Greek yogurt

INSTRUCTIONS

01 Add frozen pineapple, kale, avocado, coconut oil, coconut water in a blender and blend them until smooth and creamy.

02 When it looks smooth, then pour it into a glass and serve.

PREP TIME & SERVING

Prep time: 10 minutes
Total time: 10 minutes
Ready in about: 10 mins
No. of serve: 1

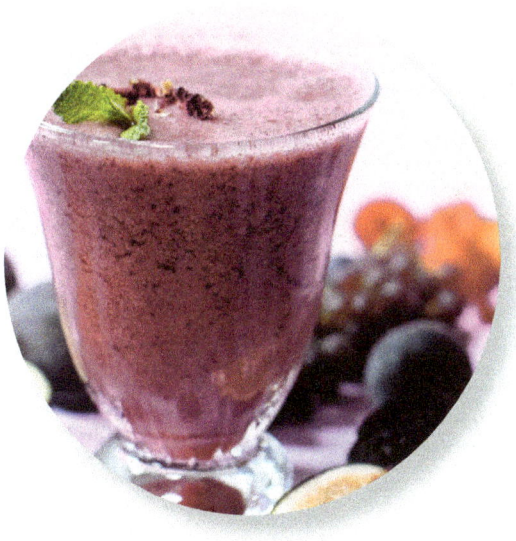

TRIPLE BERRY SMOOTHIE

ENERGY BOOSTER SMOOTHIE

INGREDIENTS

- 1 banana
- 1 cup frozen strawberries
- 1 cup frozen blackberries
- 1 cup raspberries
- 1 cup almond milk
- ½ cup Greek Yogurt

INSTRUCTIONS

01 Take a blender to add frozen strawberries, blackberries, raspberries, banana, almond milk, and Greek yogurt blend them for a minute.

02 When it looks smooth, then pour it into a glass serve.

PREP TIME & SERVING

Prep time: 5 minutes
Total time: 5 minutes
Ready in about: 5 mins
No. of serve: 1

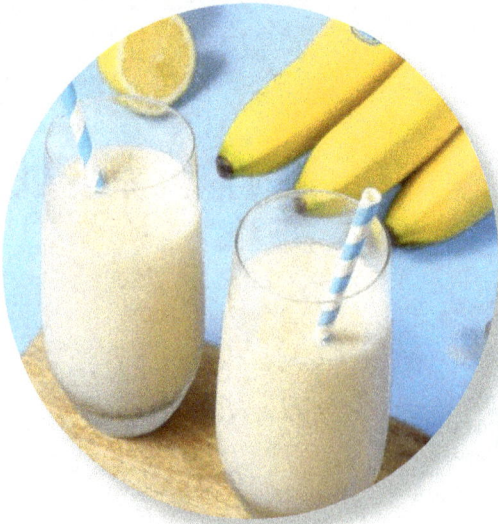

PINA COLADA ENERGY BOOST SMOOTHIE

ENERGY BOOSTER SMOOTHIE

INGREDIENTS

- 1 cup frozen pineapple
- 1 banana
- 1 cup coconut milk
- ¼ teaspoon vanilla extract

INSTRUCTIONS

01 Add frozen pineapple, banana, vanilla extract, and coconut milk in a blender and blend them until smooth.

02 When the required consistency looks, then pour it into a glass and serve.

PREP TIME & SERVING

Prep time: 5 minutes
Total time: 5 minutes
Ready in about: 5 mins
No. of serve: 1

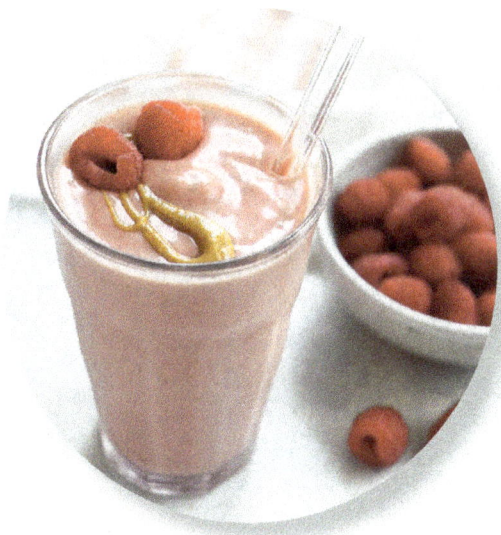

PEANUT BUTTER AND JELLY SMOOTHIE

ENERGY BOOSTER SMOOTHIE

INGREDIENTS

- 1 banana
- 2 tablespoons peanut butter
- 2 dates
- 1 cup almond milk
- ½ cup raspberries

INSTRUCTIONS

01 Use a high-speed blender and blend them for a few minutes.

02 When the required consistency is looked then pour it into a glass and serve.

PREP TIME & SERVING

Prep time: 5 minutes
Total time: 5 minutes
Ready in about: 5 mins
No. of serve: 1

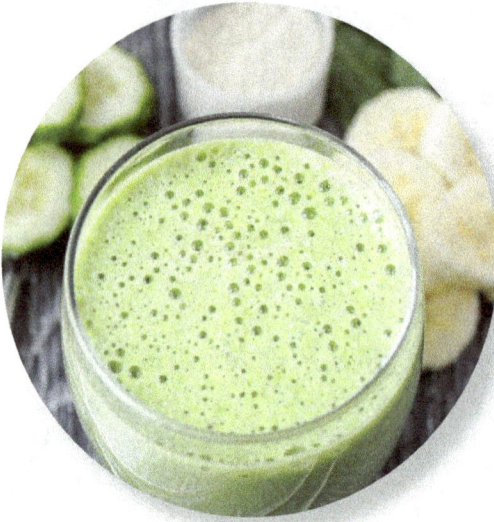

GREEN PROTEIN SMOOTHIE

ENERGY BOOSTER SMOOTHIE

INGREDIENTS

- 1 banana
- 1 cup spinach
- ½ cucumbers
- 1 scoop vanilla protein powder
- 1 cup almond milk

INSTRUCTIONS

01 Take a blender to add banana, spinach, cucumber, vanilla powder, and almond milk and blend for 1 minute.

02 Blend until it looks a smooth texture, then pour into a glass and serve.

PREP TIME & SERVING

Prep time: 4 minutes
Total time: 7 minutes
Ready in about: 7 mins
No. of serve: 1

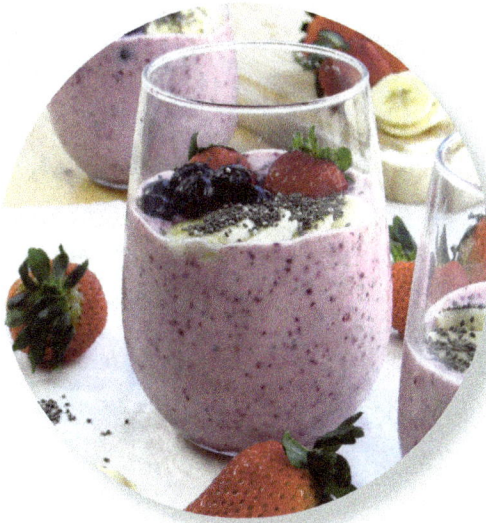

THE ENERGIZER SMOOTH-
IE

ENERGY BOOSTER SMOOTHIE

INGREDIENTS

- ½ mangos
- ½ banana
- ½ cup blueberries
- 2 tbsp chia seeds
- 1 tbsp honey
- 2 tbsp Greek Yogurt
- 3 ice cubes

INSTRUCTIONS

01 Grab a high-speed blender and blend all these ingredients.

02 Blend them well until it turns in a smooth form. If the mixture is thin, then add water as you like.

03 When the required consistency looks, then pour it into a glass. Serve

PREP TIME & SERVING

Prep time: 3 minutes
Total time: 5 minutes
Ready in about: 5 mins
No. of serve: 1

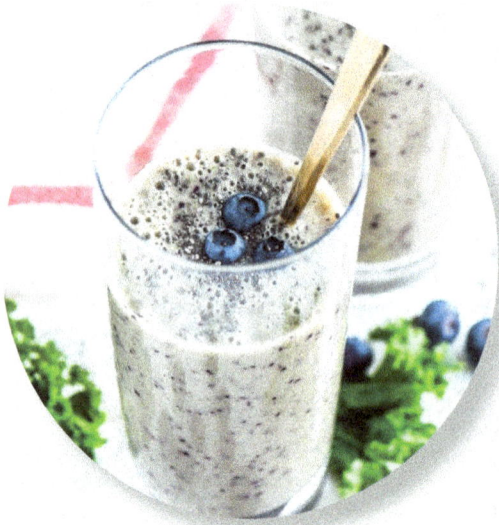

ENERGY BURST HEALTHY MORNING SMOOTHIE

ENERGY BOOSTER SMOOTHIE

INGREDIENTS

- ½ cup orange juice
- 1 banana
- 1 cup kale
- ½ cup cantaloupe
- ½ cup honey
- ½ cup frozen pineapple
- ½ cup frozen blueberries
- 1 teaspoon chia seeds
- 1 cup Greek Yogurt
- 1 cup caffeinated green tea

INSTRUCTIONS

01 Take a strong blender to add banana, frozen pineapple, frozen blueberries, orange juice, and Greek Yogurt.

02 Also, add the rest ingredients and blend them until smooth.

03 When it looks smooth, then pour it into a glass. Serve!

PREP TIME & SERVING

Prep time: 5 minutes
Total time: 5 minutes
Ready in about: 5 mins
No. of serve: 3

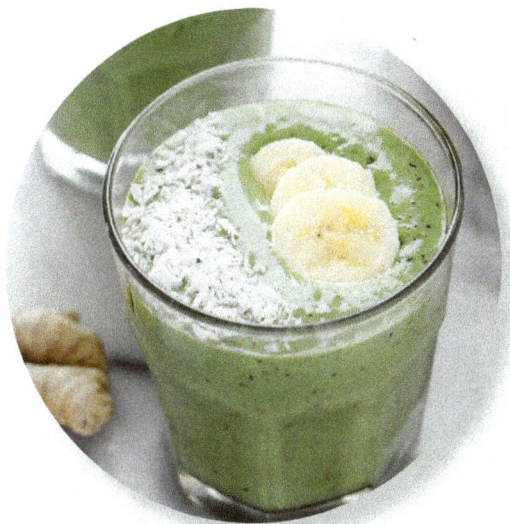

GO-GREEN ENERGIZER SMOOTHIE

ENERGY BOOSTER SMOOTHIE

INGREDIENTS

- 2 teaspoons matcha powder
- 1-2 teaspoons honey
- 2 tablespoons bee pollen
- 2 frozen bananas
- 1 piece of ginger
- 1 cup coconut milk

PREP TIME & SERVING

Prep time: 3 minutes
Total time: 5 minutes
Ready in about: 5 mins
No. of serve: 1

INSTRUCTIONS

01 Grab a high-speed blender and blend all these ingredients.

02 Blend them well until it turns in a smooth form.

03 When the required consistency looks, then pour into a glass. Serve fresh

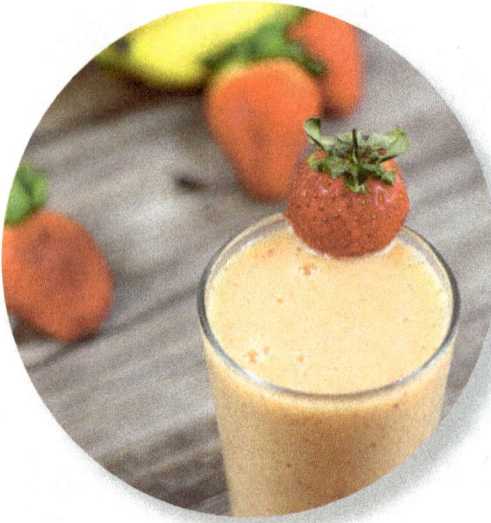

GREEK YOGURT MANGO SMOOTHIE

ENERGY BOOSTER SMOOTHIE

INGREDIENTS

- 1 cup frozen strawberries
- 1 cup frozen mango
- 1 banana
- ½ cup Greek Yogurt
- 1 cup milk
- 1 tablespoon lemon juice
- ½ cup ice

PREP TIME & SERVING

Prep time: 5 minutes
Total time: 5 minutes
Ready in about: 5 mins
No. of serve: 3

INSTRUCTIONS

01 Add frozen strawberries, mango, banana with milk, and yogurt.

02 Also, add the rest ingredients and blend them until smooth and creamy.

03 When it looks smooth, then pour it into a glass and serve right away.

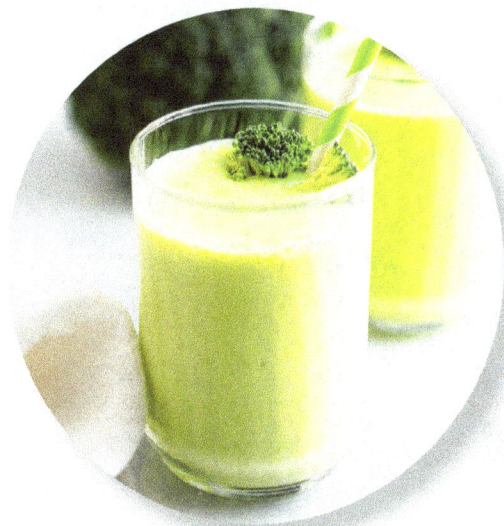

MAGIC BROCCOLI SMOOTHIE

ENERGY BOOSTER SMOOTHIE

INGREDIENTS

- ½ cup Greek Yogurt
- ½ cup water
- 1 cup chopped broccoli
- 1 large apple
- 1 banana
- 1 cup frozen pineapple

INSTRUCTIONS

01 Mix all ingredients in a high-speed blender and blend them until smooth.

02 When the required consistency looks smooth, then pour it into small glasses and serve right away.

PREP TIME & SERVING

Prep time: 3 minutes
Total time: 5 minutes
Ready in about: 5 mins
No. of serve: 1

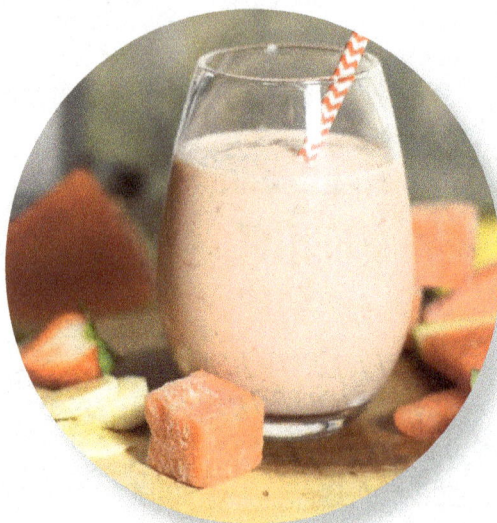

WATERMELON BANANA SMOOTHIE

ENERGY BOOSTER SMOOTHIE

INGREDIENTS

- 3 cups frozen watermelon
- 2 cups frozen strawberries
- 1 banana

INSTRUCTIONS

01 Take a blender, add frozen watermelon, strawberries, and banana blend them until smooth.

02 Pour it into glasses. Serve immediately.

PREP TIME & SERVING

Prep time: 5 minutes
Total time: 5 minutes
Ready in about: 5 mins
No. of serve: 2

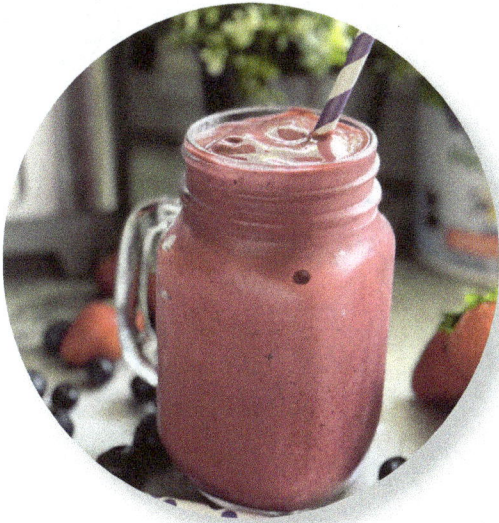

MORNING ENERGY BOOSTER SMOOTHIE

ENERGY BOOSTER SMOOTHIE

INGREDIENTS

- 3 tablespoons vanilla yogurt
- 1 cup fresh spinach
- 1 cup prune juice
- 1 cup frozen blueberries
- 6 frozen strawberries
- ½ sliced frozen peach
- 2 tablespoons flax seeds

INSTRUCTIONS

01 Use a high-speed blender and blend at high speed for 1 minute.

02 When it looks smooth, then pour it into glasses. Serve fresh.

PREP TIME & SERVING

Prep time: 7 minutes
Total time: 10 minutes
Ready in about: 10 mins
No. of serve: 2

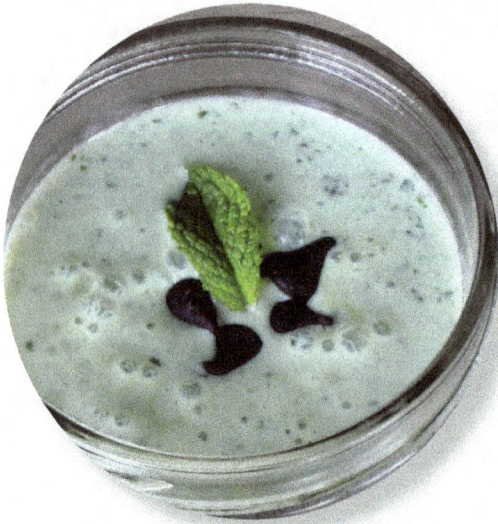

CREAMY MINT ENERGY BOOST SMOOTHIE

ENERGY BOOSTER SMOOTHIE

INGREDIENTS

- 1 frozen banana
- 1 cup chilled coconut milk
- ¼ cup avocado
- 3 pitted dates
- 1 tablespoon honey
- Handful baby spinach
- ¼ teaspoon of vanilla
- ¼ cup fresh mint leaves

INSTRUCTIONS

01 Use a high-speed blender and blend until high-speed for 1 minute.

02 When it looks smooth, then pour it into a glass. Serve fresh.

PREP TIME & SERVING

Prep time: 7 minutes
Total time: 10 minutes
Ready in about: 10 mins
No. of serve: 1

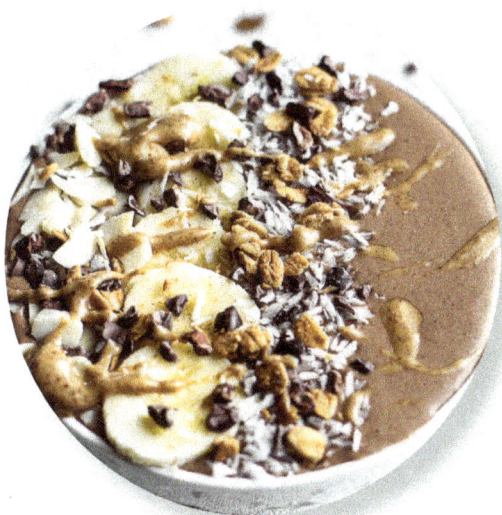

CHOCO-BANANA SMOOTHIE BOWL

ENERGY BOOSTER SMOOTHIE

INGREDIENTS

- 1 frozen banana
- ½ cup coconut milk
- 1 tablespoon cacao powder
- 1 tablespoon shredded coconut
- 1 tablespoon coconut oil
- ½ tablespoon maca powder
- 1 teaspoon vanilla
- 1 teaspoon chia seeds
- 2 dates

PREP TIME & SERVING

Prep time: 7 minutes
Total time: 10 minutes
Ready in about: 10 mins
No. of serve: 1

INSTRUCTIONS

01 Thoroughly mix all ingredients in a blender blend until for few minutes.

02 When the mixture looks smooth, then pour it into a bowl.

03 Serve right away.

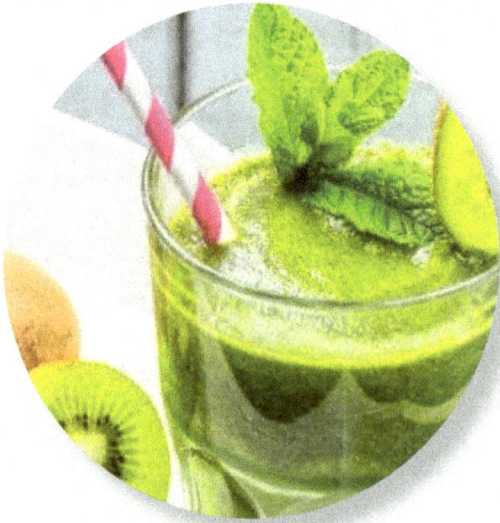

KIWI HONEYDEW ENERGY BOOSTING SMOOTHIE

ENERGY BOOSTER SMOOTHIE

INGREDIENTS

- 1 banana
- ¼ cup of a large honeydew
- 3 kiwis
- 1 cup almond milk
- 1 tablespoon chia seeds (optional)
- 4 ice cubes
- 1 cup spinach leaves

INSTRUCTIONS

01 Take a high-speed blender and add banana, honeydew, kiwis, almond milk, spinach, and ice cubes blend for few minutes.

02 When the required consistency is looking smooth, then pour it into glasses and serve fresh.

PREP TIME & SERVING

Prep time: 10 minutes
Total time: 10 minutes
Ready in about: 10 mins
No. of serve: 1

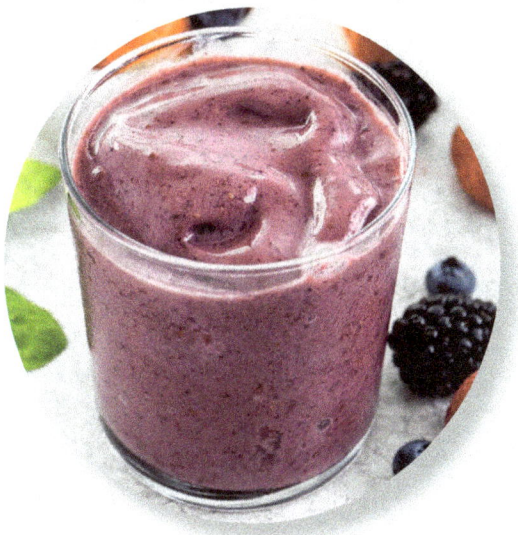

ENERGY BOOSTING BERRY BLEND SMOOTHIE

ENERGY BOOSTER SMOOTHIE

INGREDIENTS

- 2 cups baby spinach
- 1 cucumber
- ½ cup frozen mixed berries
- ½ cup frozen raspberries
- 1 cup almond milk
- Stevia, to taste

PREP TIME & SERVING

Prep time: 5 minutes
Total time: 5 minutes
Ready in about: 5 mins
No. of serve: 1

INSTRUCTIONS

01 Grab a strong blender and adds the entire ingredients to it.

02 Blend them for a minute until they turn into a smooth form.

03 Pour it into a smoothie jar and serve cold.

CPSIA information can be obtained
at www.ICGtesting.com
Printed in the USA
BVHW091427300421
606211BV00006B/1001